STONEWELL HEALING PRESS

HOW TO USE THIS BOOK

Think of this book as your health companion — a place to finally put the pieces together. Symptoms rarely happen in isolation. They show up with timing, patterns, triggers, and shifts that are easy to miss until they're written down.

Here's how to make the most of these pages:

- **Track regularly.** You don't need perfect entries — you just need honest ones. A few words are enough.
- **Note the small things.** A food that didn't sit right. A feeling of pressure. A bad night of sleep. A spike in anxiety. These details matter.
- **Use the guided pages to explore deeper.** Medications, flares, digestion, mental health, pain, energy — the more you record, the clearer your patterns become.
- **Bring this book with you.** It can help you advocate for yourself, remember timelines, and communicate your experience without scrambling.
- **Review your notes often.** You may notice patterns long before a provider does.

There's no right way to fill this out — only the way that helps you feel understood, supported, and one step closer to answers.

THE LONG ROAD TO
A DIAGNOSIS

Getting answers isn't usually a straight line. It's a winding road with stops, clues, patterns, and breakthroughs. This book is not just a companion on that journey—it is the tool that turns confusion into clarity.

1 Getting Sick

Symptoms begin. You search online, ask around, try home remedies, or wait it out. Nothing adds up, and nothing fully explains what you're experiencing.

2 New/Persistent Symptoms

Episodes repeat. New symptoms show up. You start to realize this isn't going away on its own.

3 No Answers

You don't find the answers you need. You don't receive answers despite appointments with your providers or the information you find.

5 Finding Healing

This roadmap carries you toward your diagnosis. If you don't get answers right away, this book helps you advocate for more testing, referrals, or second opinions. Either way, you move forward, not in circles.

4 Searching For A Diagnosis

This is where you take back control. You begin tracking everything in this book — patterns, triggers, daily impact, symptom timing, lab results, and questions for your doctor. This is the turning point. Your observations become organized, visible, and impossible to overlook.

IMPORTANT NOTES

_____

_____

_____

_____

_____

_____

_____

_____

_____

_____

_____

_____

_____

_____

_____

_____

_____

SYMPTOM SNAPSHOT
YOUR BASELINE

Before you begin tracking day-to-day changes, use this page to create a clear picture of what you're experiencing right now. This becomes your personal "before" — the starting point you and your healthcare provider can return to as symptoms evolve or patterns become clearer.

Fill it out as fully as you can. If you're unsure about something, note that instead.

Top Current Symptoms	When It Started (after surgery, childhood, etc.)	Severity (1-10)	Frequency (hourly, weekly, etc.)
○ _____	_____	_____	_____
○ _____	_____	_____	_____
○ _____	_____	_____	_____
○ _____	_____	_____	_____
○ _____	_____	_____	_____
○ _____	_____	_____	_____
○ _____	_____	_____	_____
○ _____	_____	_____	_____
○ _____	_____	_____	_____
○ _____	_____	_____	_____

Suspected Triggers	What Helps
○ _____	_____
○ _____	_____
○ _____	_____
○ _____	_____
○ _____	_____
○ _____	_____
○ _____	_____
○ _____	_____

IMPORTANT NOTES

SYMPTOM SNAPSHOT
YOUR BASELINE

Before you begin tracking day-to-day changes, use this page to create a clear picture of what you're experiencing right now. This becomes your personal "before" — the starting point you and your healthcare provider can return to as symptoms evolve or patterns become clearer.
Fill it out as fully as you can. If you're unsure about something, note that instead.

Top Current Symptoms	When It Started (after surgery, childhood, etc.)	Severity (1-10)	Frequency (hourly, weekly, etc.)
○			
○			
○			
○			
○			
○			
○			
○			
○			
○			

Suspected Triggers	What Helps
○	
○	
○	
○	
○	
○	
○	
○	

IMPORTANT NOTES

TIMELINE OF SYMPTOMS & FLARES
YOUR BASELINE

Keeping a timeline helps you see patterns that might be invisible day-to-day. By mapping symptoms alongside major events in your life, you can start to notice triggers, connections, and cycles that are often missed in conversation or appointment notes.

Use this page to track when symptoms first appeared, when they worsened, and anything else that might be linked — physical, emotional, or environmental.

Symptom/Flare	Duration	Trigger	Frequency
○ _____	_____	_____	_____
○ _____	_____	_____	_____
○ _____	_____	_____	_____
○ _____	_____	_____	_____
○ _____	_____	_____	_____
○ _____	_____	_____	_____
○ _____	_____	_____	_____
○ _____	_____	_____	_____
○ _____	_____	_____	_____
○ _____	_____	_____	_____

What Makes It Worse	What Helps
_____	_____
_____	_____
_____	_____
_____	_____
_____	_____
_____	_____
_____	_____

IMPORTANT NOTES

_____
_____
_____
_____
_____
_____
_____
_____
_____
_____
_____
_____
_____
_____
_____
_____
_____
_____
_____
_____
_____

WHAT YOU'VE ALREADY TRIED
YOUR BASELINE

Understanding what you've already experimented with — treatments, routines, medications, lifestyle shifts — helps you and your healthcare provider avoid repetition and move toward answers more efficiently. This page gives you a clear record of what's been helpful, what hasn't, and what made things worse.

Medications You've Tried	Dose	Result

Lifestyle Changes You've Tried	Result

IMPORTANT NOTES

WHAT YOU'VE ALREADY TRIED
YOUR BASELINE

Understanding what you've already experimented with — treatments, routines, medications, lifestyle shifts — helps you and your healthcare provider avoid repetition and move toward answers more efficiently. This page gives you a clear record of what's been helpful, what hasn't, and what made things worse.

Dietary Changes	Length Of Trial	Result
_____	_____	_____
_____	_____	_____
_____	_____	_____
_____	_____	_____
_____	_____	_____
_____	_____	_____
_____	_____	_____

Notes:

_____

_____

_____

_____

_____

WHAT YOU'VE ALREADY TRIED
YOUR BASELINE

TEST

APPROX DATE

NOTES

TEST

APPROX DATE

NOTES

TEST

APPROX DATE

NOTES

TEST

APPROX DATE

NOTES

WHAT YOU'VE ALREADY TRIED
YOUR BASELINE

WHAT YOU KNOW FOR SURE

1.

2.

3.

4.

5.

6.

THOUGHTS & REFLECTIONS

WHAT YOU'VE ALREADY TRIED
YOUR BASELINE

WHAT MADE THINGS WORSE

1.

2.

3.

4.

5.

6.

THOUGHTS & REFLECTIONS

WHAT YOU'VE ALREADY TRIED
YOUR BASELINE

WHAT I'M UNSURE ABOUT

1.

2.

3.

4.

5.

6.

THOUGHTS & REFLECTIONS

IMPORTANT NOTES

MY WORST DAYS
YOUR BASELINE

Describe symptoms, pain levels, mood, energy, digestion, mental clarity, mobility, etc.

What I Struggle To Do On My Worst Days

	LOW	HIGH
FATIGUE	o—o—o—o—o	
HEADACHE	o—o—o—o—o	
NAUSEA	o—o—o—o—o	
GI UPSET	o—o—o—o—o	
DIFFICULTY SLEEPING	o—o—o—o—o	
MUSCLE TENSION	o—o—o—o—o	
DIZZINESS/LIGHTHEADEDNESS	o—o—o—o—o	
WALKING/MOBILITY	o—o—o—o—o	
STANDING	o—o—o—o—o	
EATING NORMALLY	o—o—o—o—o	
EATING	o o o o o	
DRINKING/SWALLOWING	o—o—o—o—o	
TALKING/SOCIALIZING	o—o—o—o—o	
LEAVING THE HOUSE	o—o—o—o—o	
CHRONIC PAIN	o—o—o—o—o	
OTHER:	o—o—o—o—o	
OTHER:	o—o—o—o—o	
OTHER:	o—o—o—o—o	
OTHER:	o—o—o—o—o	
OTHER:	o—o—o—o—o	

What usually triggers or leads to a worst day

○ _____
○ _____
○ _____
○ _____
○ _____

How Long Do These Episodes Typically Last

How Often Do These Days Occur

Are These Days/Episodes

RANDOM ☐   REGULAR ☐   SELDOM ☐

Daily Function

ABILITY TO WORK (1–10)	_____
SOCIAL INTERACTIONS (1–10)	_____
CONCENTRATION (1–10)	_____
ENERGY / MOTIVATION (1–10)	_____
PHYSICAL ACTIVITY (1–10)	_____

Medication Effectiveness

O———O———O———O———O
LOW   HIGH

Medication Impact

O———O———O———O
NEGATIVE   POSITIVE

IMPORTANT NOTES

MY BEST DAYS
YOUR BASELINE

Describe symptoms, pain levels, mood, energy, digestion, mental clarity, mobility, etc.

What Symptoms I have on my best days

	LOW				HIGH
FATIGUE	O—O—O—O—O
HEADACHE	O—O—O—O—O
NAUSEA	O—O—O—O—O
GI UPSET	O—O—O—O—O
DIFFICULTY SLEEPING	O—O—O—O—O
MUSCLE TENSION	O—O—O—O—O
DIZZINESS/LIGHTHEADEDNESS	O—O—O—O—O
WALKING/MOBILITY	O—O—O—O—O
STANDING	O—O—O—O—O
EATING NORMALLY	O—O—O—O—O
EATING	O O O O O
DRINKING/SWALLOWING	O—O—O—O—O
TALKING/SOCIALIZING	O—O—O—O—O
LEAVING THE HOUSE	O—O—O—O—O
CHRONIC PAIN	O—O—O—O—O
OTHER:	O—O—O—O—O
OTHER:	O—O—O—O—O
OTHER:	O—O—O—O—O
OTHER:	O—O—O—O—O
OTHER:	O—O—O—O—O

Daily Function

ABILITY TO WORK (1–10)   _____

SOCIAL INTERACTIONS (1–10)   _____

CONCENTRATION (1–10)   _____

ENERGY / MOTIVATION (1–10)   _____

PHYSICAL ACTIVITY (1–10)   _____

What I'm able to do on my best days

O _____

O _____

O _____

O _____

O _____

How many good days do you have in a row (usually)

How Often Do These Days Occur

Are These Days

RANDOM ☐   REGULAR ☐   SELDOM ☐

What tends to support my best days

O _____

O _____

O _____

O _____

O _____

EMOTIONAL TOLL
IMPACT OF SYMPTOMS

Use this space to describe how your physical symptoms impact your emotional well-being. Consider: frustration, fear, sadness, irritability, overwhelm, discouragement, embarrassment, or feeling misunderstood.

HOW HAVE YOUR SYMPTOMS AFFECTED YOUR EMOTIONAL STATE?

_____

_____

_____

_____

_____

_____

_____

_____

_____

_____

_____

_____

_____

EMOTIONAL TOLL
IMPACT OF SYMPTOMS

Chronic or unexplained symptoms often lead to fear of the unknown, worry about flare-ups, and stress related to unpredictability.

WHAT WORRIES OR STRESSES HAVE COME UP BECAUSE OF YOUR HEALTH?

_____

_____

_____

_____

_____

_____

_____

_____

_____

_____

_____

_____

_____

_____

EMOTIONAL TOLL
IMPACT OF SYMPTOMS

Symptoms can strain connections, limit activities, or affect communication.
This can have major impacts on relationships and social life.

HOW HAVE YOUR SYMPTOMS AFFECTED YOUR RELATIONSHIPS,
SOCIAL INTERACTIONS, OR SUPPORT SYSTEM?

_____

_____

_____

_____

_____

_____

_____

_____

_____

_____

_____

_____

EMOTIONAL TOLL
IMPACT OF SYMPTOMS

Your condition may interfere with focus, energy, routines, obligations, or responsibilities. This can impact your work, parenting, and overall daily functioning.

WHAT CHALLENGES HAVE YOUR SYMPTOMS CREATED IN YOUR DAILY RESPONSIBILITIES?

_____

_____

_____

_____

_____

_____

_____

_____

_____

_____

_____

_____

_____

_____

EMOTIONAL TOLL
IMPACT OF SYMPTOMS

Your condition may interfere with focus, energy, routines, obligations, or responsibilities. This can impact your work, parenting, and overall daily functioning.

WHAT CHALLENGES HAVE YOUR SYMPTOMS CREATED IN YOUR DAILY RESPONSIBILITIES?

_____

_____

_____

_____

_____

_____

_____

_____

_____

_____

_____

_____

_____

_____

EMOTIONAL TOLL
IMPACT OF SYMPTOMS

Many people feel as though their doctor's don't understand the extent or impact of their condition. Use this area to express things that are difficult to say in appointments but are essential to your lived experience.

WHAT DO YOU WISH YOUR DOCTOR UNDERSTOOD ABOUT THE IMPACT YOUR SYMPTOMS HAVE ON YOUR LIFE?

_____

_____

_____

_____

_____

_____

_____

_____

_____

_____

_____

_____

_____

_____

_____

_____

EMOTIONAL TOLL
IMPACT OF SYMPTOMS

Use these bullet points to clearly explain how your symptoms affect your ability to function day-to-day. Bring this page to your appointments or review it with your current healthcare provider or any new providers.

WHAT DO YOU WISH YOUR DOCTOR UNDERSTOOD ABOUT THE IMPACT YOUR SYMPTOMS HAVE ON YOUR LIFE?

1. _____

2. _____

3. _____

4. _____

5. _____

6. _____

7. _____

EMOTIONAL TOLL
IMPACT OF SYMPTOMS

Use these bullet points to clearly explain how your symptoms affect your ability to function day-to-day. Bring this page to your appointments or review it with your current healthcare provider or any new providers.

WHAT DO YOU WISH YOUR DOCTOR UNDERSTOOD ABOUT THE IMPACT YOUR SYMPTOMS HAVE ON YOUR LIFE?

1.

2.

3.

4.

5.

6.

7.

EMOTIONAL TOLL
IMPACT OF SYMPTOMS

Use these bullet points to clearly explain how your symptoms affect your ability to function day-to-day. Bring this page to your appointments or review it with your current healthcare provider or any new providers.

WHAT DO YOU WISH YOUR DOCTOR UNDERSTOOD ABOUT THE IMPACT YOUR SYMPTOMS HAVE ON YOUR LIFE?

Physical Functioning

FATIGUE IMPACTING DAILY TASKS ☐
PAIN INTERFERING DAILY LIFE ☐
REDUCED STAMINA ☐
TROUBLE COMPLETING HYGIENE ☐
DIFFICULTY STANDING, WALKING, ☐
LIFTING, OR MOVING NORMALLY

Cognitive Functioning

BRAIN FOG ☐
DIFFICULTY CONCENTRATING ☐
MEMORY ISSUES ☐
BLACKOUT/DISASOCIATION ☐
TROUBLE MAKING DECISIONS OR ☐
PROCESSING INFORMATION

Sleep & Energy

WAKING UNREFRESHED ☐
NIGHT TERRORS ☐
WORSED PAIN AT NIGHT ☐
DAYTIME EXHAUSTION ☐
TROUBLE FALLING ASLEEP OR ☐
STAYING ASLEEP

Emotional Impact

INCREASED STRESS OR ANXIETY ☐
SOCIAL WITHDRAWAL OR ISOLATION ☐
DEPRESSION/EXCESSIVE SADNESS ☐
ANXIETY/PANIC ☐
MOOD SWINGS ☐

Symptom Patterns Affecting Life

UNPREDICTABLE FLARE-UPS ☐
SYMPTOMS TRIGGERED BY FOOD ☐
SYMPTOMS TRIGGERED BY STRESS ☐
SYMPTOMS TRIGGERED BY ACTIVITY ☐
WORSENING SYMPTOMS AT ☐
SPECIFIC TIMES OF DAY

Limitations & Safety Concerns

UNABLE TO DRIVE SAFELY ☐
INCREASED RISK OF FALLS OR ACCIDENTS ☐
INABILITY TO CARE FOR SELF ☐
INABILITY TO CARE FOR OTHERS ☐
DIFFICULTY WORKING WITH ☐
MACHINERY
DANGER TO SELF ☐
DANGER TO OTHERS ☐

IMPORTANT NOTES

NEW WEEK CHECK-IN
PATTERNS & NOTES

How Did Last Week Go Overall?   ○———○———○———○———○

MUCH WORSE   MUCH BETTER

Any Clear Patterns Or Triggers?   New Things You're Trying This Week

○ _____   ○ _____
○ _____   ○ _____
○ _____   ○ _____
○ _____   ○ _____
○ _____   ○ _____

Changes To Medication/Supplements?   YES ☐   NO ☐

NOTE: _____

Changes To Treatment/Therapies?   YES ☐   NO ☐

NOTE: _____

Emotional & Mental Health Check-In

HOW ARE YOU FEELING HEADING INTO THIS WEEK? ANYTHING WEIGHING ON YOU?

_____

_____

_____

_____

_____

_____

DAILY SYMPTOM TRACKER

Date:

Sleep
QUALITY (1-10) _____ LENGTH _____

Flare Status
SUDDEN ☐ TRIGGERED ☐
SLOW BUILDING ☐ RANDOM ☐

NO FLARE ○ ○ ○ ○ ○ SEVERE FLAIR
MILD MODERATE

Weather
HOT ☐ DRY ☐ HUMID ☐
RAIN ☐ STORM ☐ COLD ☐

SUSPECTED TRIGGER _____

Today's Symptoms

	LOW	HIGH
FEVER	○—○—○—○—○	
FATIGUE	○—○—○—○—○	

Systemic

DIZZINESS ☐ NIGHT SWEATS ☐
WEIGHT CHANGE ☐ FLUE-LIKE ☐
CHILLS ☐ BRAIN FOG ☐

Pain & Inflammation

JOINT PAIN ☐ JOINT SWELLING ☐
STIFFNESS ☐ MUSCLE ACHES ☐
WEAKNESS ☐ BACK PAIN ☐
NERVE PAIN ☐ MIGRAINES ☐

Thyroid-like

TREMORS ☐ HEART PALPITATIONS ☐
HEAT/COLD SENSITITVITY ☐ WEIGHT SHIFT ☐
CHILLS ☐ NECK PAIN ☐

Skin, Hair & Nails

RASH ☐ REDNESS/FLUSHING ☐
HIVES ☐ SENSITITY TO SUN ☐
ITCHING ☐ BRITTLE NAILS ☐
HAIR LOSS ☐ DRY SKIN ☐

Respiratory

CHEST PAIN ☐ CHRONIC COUGH ☐
SHORTNESS OF BREATH ☐

Kidneys

FOAMY URINE ☐ SWELLING IN LEGS / ANKLES ☐
DARK URINE ☐ BLOODY URINE ☐

Digestive / GI

NAUSEA ☐ STOMACH PAINS ☐
VOMITING ☐ FOOD REACTIONS ☐
DIARRHEA ☐ APPETITE LOSS ☐
CONSTIPATION ☐ BLOATING ☐

Vascular

NUMB FINGERS/TOES ☐ RAYNAUD'S COLOR CHANGES ☐

DAILY SYMPTOM TRACKER

Date:

Stress Level

O—O—O—O—O
LOW   HIGH

Pain's Impact On Today's Function
Today pain affected my ability to:

DRIVE ☐   WORK ☐   SOCIALIZE ☐

COOK ☐   LIFT/CARRY ☐   LEAVE THE HOUSE ☐

WALK ☐   CARE FOR SELF ☐   SIT/LAY DOWN ☐

Symptom Changes Throughout The Day

CONSISTENT ☐   WORSE AT NIGHT ☐

COMES IN WAVES ☐   PAIN FLARE ☐

WORSE IN MORNING ☐

Notes

_____

_____

_____

_____

_____

_____

_____

_____

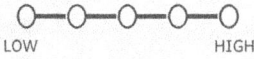

Today's Water Intake

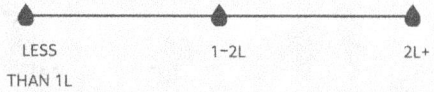

◆———————◆———————◆
LESS THAN 1L   1–2L   2L+

Food & Immune Response

DID YOU EAT ANYTHING NEW TODAY?

YES ☐   NO ☐

Impact On Symptoms

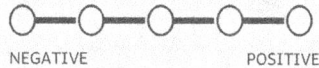

O—O—O—O—O
NEGATIVE   POSITIVE

Notes

_____

_____

_____

_____

_____

_____

Activity Overview

REST DAY ☐   LIGHT MOVEMENT ☐

MODERATE ACTIVITY ☐   HEAVY ACTIVITY ☐

Effect On Pain

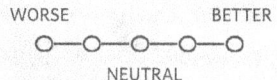

         WORSE   BETTER

O—O—O—O—O

        NEUTRAL

DAILY SYMPTOM TRACKER

Date:

Sleep QUALITY (1-10) _____ LENGTH _____

Flare Status
SUDDEN ☐ TRIGGERED ☐
SLOW BUILDING ☐ RANDOM ☐

Weather
HOT ☐ DRY ☐ HUMID ☐
RAIN ☐ STORM ☐ COLD ☐

NO FLARE ○ ○ ○ ○ ○ SEVERE FLAIR
MILD MODERATE

SUSPECTED TRIGGER _____

Today's Symptoms

Systemic

	LOW	HIGH
FEVER	○—○—○—○—○	
FATIGUE	○—○—○—○—○	

DIZZINESS ☐ NIGHT SWEATS ☐
WEIGHT CHANGE ☐ FLUE-LIKE ☐
CHILLS ☐ BRAIN FOG ☐

Pain & Inflammation

JOINT PAIN ☐ JOINT SWELLING ☐
STIFFNESS ☐ MUSCLE ACHES ☐
WEAKNESS ☐ BACK PAIN ☐
NERVE PAIN ☐ MIGRAINES ☐

Thyroid-like

TREMORS ☐ HEART PALPITATIONS ☐
HEAT/COLD SENSITITVITY ☐ WEIGHT SHIFT ☐
CHILLS ☐ NECK PAIN ☐

Skin, Hair & Nails

RASH ☐ REDNESS/FLUSHING ☐
HIVES ☐ SENSITITY TO SUN ☐
ITCHING ☐ BRITTLE NAILS ☐
HAIR LOSS ☐ DRY SKIN ☐

Respiratory

CHEST PAIN ☐ CHRONIC COUGH ☐
SHORTNESS OF BREATH ☐

Kidneys

FOAMY URINE ☐ SWELLING IN LEGS / ANKLES ☐
DARK URINE ☐ BLOODY URINE ☐

Digestive / GI

NAUSEA ☐ STOMACH PAINS ☐
VOMITING ☐ FOOD REACTIONS ☐
DIARRHEA ☐ APPETITE LOSS ☐
CONSTIPATION ☐ BLOATING ☐

Vascular

NUMB FINGERS/TOES ☐ RAYNAUD'S COLOR CHANGES ☐

DAILY SYMPTOM TRACKER

Date:

Stress Level

O—O—O—O—O
LOW   HIGH

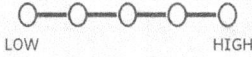

Pain's Impact On Today's Function
Today pain affected my ability to:

DRIVE ☐	WORK ☐	SOCIALIZE ☐
COOK ☐	LIFT/CARRY ☐	LEAVE THE HOUSE ☐
WALK ☐	CARE FOR SELF ☐	SIT/LAY DOWN ☐

Symptom Changes Throughout The Day

CONSISTENT ☐	WORSE AT NIGHT ☐
COMES IN WAVES ☐	PAIN FLARE ☐
WORSE IN MORNING ☐	

Notes

_____
_____
_____
_____
_____
_____
_____

Today's Water Intake

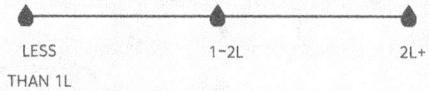

◆————◆————◆
LESS THAN 1L   1–2L   2L+

Food & Immune Response

DID YOU EAT ANYTHING NEW TODAY?
YES ☐   NO ☐

Impact On Symptoms

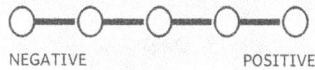

O—O—O—O—O
NEGATIVE   POSITIVE

Notes

_____
_____
_____
_____
_____
_____

Activity Overview

REST DAY ☐	LIGHT MOVEMENT ☐
MODERATE ACTIVITY ☐	HEAVY ACTIVITY ☐

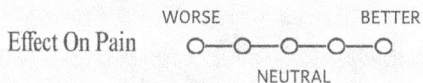

WORSE   BETTER
Effect On Pain   O—O—O—O—O
NEUTRAL

DAILY SYMPTOM TRACKER

Date:

Sleep QUALITY (1-10) _____ LENGTH _____

Flare Status
SUDDEN ☐ TRIGGERED ☐
SLOW BUILDING ☐ RANDOM ☐

NO FLARE ○ ○ ○ ○ ○ SEVERE FLAIR
MILD MODERATE

Weather
HOT ☐ DRY ☐ HUMID ☐
RAIN ☐ STORM ☐ COLD ☐

SUSPECTED TRIGGER _____

Today's Symptoms

Systemic

	LOW	HIGH
FEVER	○—○—○—○—○	
FATIGUE	○—○—○—○—○	

DIZZINESS ☐   NIGHT SWEATS ☐
WEIGHT CHANGE ☐   FLUE-LIKE ☐
CHILLS ☐   BRAIN FOG ☐

Pain & Inflammation

JOINT PAIN ☐   JOINT SWELLING ☐
STIFFNESS ☐   MUSCLE ACHES ☐
WEAKNESS ☐   BACK PAIN ☐
NERVE PAIN ☐   MIGRAINES ☐

Thyroid-like

TREMORS ☐   HEART PALPITATIONS ☐
HEAT/COLD SENSITITVITY ☐   WEIGHT SHIFT ☐
CHILLS ☐   NECK PAIN ☐

Skin, Hair & Nails

RASH ☐   REDNESS/FLUSHING ☐
HIVES ☐   SENSITITITY TO SUN ☐
ITCHING ☐   BRITTLE NAILS ☐
HAIR LOSS ☐   DRY SKIN ☐

Respiratory

CHEST PAIN ☐   CHRONIC COUGH ☐
SHORTNESS OF BREATH ☐

Kidneys

FOAMY URINE ☐   SWELLING IN LEGS / ANKLES ☐
DARK URINE ☐   BLOODY URINE ☐

Digestive / GI

NAUSEA ☐   STOMACH PAINS ☐
VOMITING ☐   FOOD REACTIONS ☐
DIARRHEA ☐   APPETITE LOSS ☐
CONSTIPATION ☐   BLOATING ☐

Vascular

NUMB FINGERS/TOES ☐   RAYNAUD'S COLOR CHANGES ☐

DAILY SYMPTOM TRACKER

Date:

Stress Level O—O—O—O—O
            LOW   HIGH

Pain's Impact On Today's Function
Today pain affected my ability to:

DRIVE ☐   WORK ☐   SOCIALIZE ☐

COOK ☐   LIFT/CARRY ☐   LEAVE THE HOUSE ☐

WALK ☐   CARE FOR SELF ☐   SIT/LAY DOWN ☐

Symptom Changes Throughout The Day

CONSISTENT ☐   WORSE AT NIGHT ☐

COMES IN WAVES ☐   PAIN FLARE ☐

WORSE IN MORNING ☐

Notes

_____

_____

_____

_____

_____

_____

_____

Today's Water Intake

◆————————◆————————◆

LESS THAN 1L   1-2L   2L+

Food & Immune Response

DID YOU EAT ANYTHING NEW TODAY?

YES ☐   NO ☐

Impact On Symptoms

O—O—O—O—O

NEGATIVE   POSITIVE

Notes

_____

_____

_____

_____

_____

_____

Activity Overview

REST DAY ☐   LIGHT MOVEMENT ☐

MODERATE ACTIVITY ☐   HEAVY ACTIVITY ☐

             WORSE   BETTER

Effect On Pain   O—O—O—O—O

                      NEUTRAL

DAILY SYMPTOM TRACKER

Date:

Sleep	QUALITY (1-10) ____ LENGTH ____

Flare Status

SUDDEN ☐	TRIGGERED ☐
SLOW BUILDING ☐	RANDOM ☐

NO FLARE ○ ○ ○ ○ ○ SEVERE FLAIR

MILD   MODERATE

SUSPECTED TRIGGER _____

Weather

HOT ☐   DRY ☐   HUMID ☐
RAIN ☐   STORM ☐   COLD ☐

Today's Symptoms

	LOW	HIGH
FEVER	○—○—○—○—○	
FATIGUE	○—○—○—○—○	

Systemic

DIZZINESS ☐	NIGHT SWEATS ☐
WEIGHT CHANGE ☐	FLUE-LIKE ☐
CHILLS ☐	BRAIN FOG ☐

Pain & Inflammation

JOINT PAIN ☐	JOINT SWELLING ☐
STIFFNESS ☐	MUSCLE ACHES ☐
WEAKNESS ☐	BACK PAIN ☐
NERVE PAIN ☐	MIGRAINES ☐

Thyroid-like

TREMORS ☐	HEART PALPITATIONS ☐
HEAT/COLD SENSITITVITY ☐	WEIGHT SHIFT ☐
CHILLS ☐	NECK PAIN ☐

Skin, Hair & Nails

RASH ☐	REDNESS/FLUSHING ☐
HIVES ☐	SENSITITY TO SUN ☐
ITCHING ☐	BRITTLE NAILS ☐
HAIR LOSS ☐	DRY SKIN ☐

Respiratory

CHEST PAIN ☐	CHRONIC COUGH ☐
SHORTNESS OF BREATH ☐	

Kidneys

FOAMY URINE ☐	SWELLING IN LEGS / ANKLES ☐
DARK URINE ☐	BLOODY URINE ☐

Digestive / GI

NAUSEA ☐	STOMACH PAINS ☐
VOMITING ☐	FOOD REACTIONS ☐
DIARRHEA ☐	APPETITE LOSS ☐
CONSTIPATION ☐	BLOATING ☐

Vascular

NUMB FINGERS/TOES ☐	RAYNAUD'S COLOR CHANGES ☐

DAILY SYMPTOM TRACKER

Date:

Stress Level

O—O—O—O—O
LOW   HIGH

Pain's Impact On Today's Function

Today pain affected my ability to:

DRIVE ☐   WORK ☐   SOCIALIZE ☐

COOK ☐   LIFT/CARRY ☐   LEAVE THE HOUSE ☐

WALK ☐   CARE FOR SELF ☐   SIT/LAY DOWN ☐

Symptom Changes Throughout The Day

CONSISTENT ☐   WORSE AT NIGHT ☐

COMES IN WAVES ☐   PAIN FLARE ☐

WORSE IN MORNING ☐

Notes

_____

_____

_____

_____

_____

_____

_____

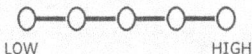

Today's Water Intake

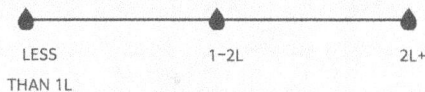

LESS THAN 1L   1–2L   2L+

Food & Immune Response

DID YOU EAT ANYTHING NEW TODAY?

YES ☐   NO ☐

Impact On Symptoms

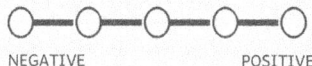

O—O—O—O—O
NEGATIVE   POSITIVE

Notes

_____

_____

_____

_____

_____

_____

Activity Overview

REST DAY ☐   LIGHT MOVEMENT ☐

MODERATE ACTIVITY ☐   HEAVY ACTIVITY ☐

Effect On Pain
WORSE   BETTER
O—O—O—O—O
NEUTRAL

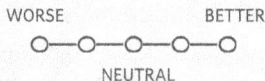

DAILY SYMPTOM TRACKER

Date:

Sleep QUALITY (1-10) _____ LENGTH _____

Flare Status
SUDDEN ☐ TRIGGERED ☐
SLOW BUILDING ☐ RANDOM ☐

NO FLARE ○ ○ ○ ○ ○ SEVERE FLAIR
MILD   MODERATE

SUSPECTED TRIGGER _____

Weather
HOT ☐ DRY ☐ HUMID ☐
RAIN ☐ STORM ☐ COLD ☐

Today's Symptoms

Systemic

	LOW	HIGH
FEVER	○—○—○—○—○	
FATIGUE	○—○—○—○—○	

DIZZINESS ☐ NIGHT SWEATS ☐
WEIGHT CHANGE ☐ FLUE-LIKE ☐
CHILLS ☐ BRAIN FOG ☐

Pain & Inflammation

JOINT PAIN ☐ JOINT SWELLING ☐
STIFFNESS ☐ MUSCLE ACHES ☐
WEAKNESS ☐ BACK PAIN ☐
NERVE PAIN ☐ MIGRAINES ☐

Thyroid-like

TREMORS ☐ HEART PALPITATIONS ☐
HEAT/COLD SENSITITVITY ☐ WEIGHT SHIFT ☐
CHILLS ☐ NECK PAIN ☐

Skin, Hair & Nails

RASH ☐ REDNESS/FLUSHING ☐
HIVES ☐ SENSITITY TO SUN ☐
ITCHING ☐ BRITTLE NAILS ☐
HAIR LOSS ☐ DRY SKIN ☐

Respiratory

CHEST PAIN ☐ CHRONIC COUGH ☐
SHORTNESS OF BREATH ☐

Kidneys

FOAMY URINE ☐ SWELLING IN LEGS / ANKLES ☐
DARK URINE ☐ BLOODY URINE ☐

Digestive / GI

NAUSEA ☐ STOMACH PAINS ☐
VOMITING ☐ FOOD REACTIONS ☐
DIARRHEA ☐ APPETITE LOSS ☐
CONSTIPATION ☐ BLOATING ☐

Vascular

NUMB FINGERS/TOES ☐ RAYNAUD'S COLOR CHANGES ☐

DAILY SYMPTOM TRACKER

Date:

Stress Level

O—O—O—O—O

LOW   HIGH

Pain's Impact On Today's Function
Today pain affected my ability to:

DRIVE ☐   WORK ☐   SOCIALIZE ☐

COOK ☐   LIFT/CARRY ☐   LEAVE THE HOUSE ☐

WALK ☐   CARE FOR SELF ☐   SIT/LAY DOWN ☐

Symptom Changes Throughout The Day

CONSISTENT ☐   WORSE AT NIGHT ☐

COMES IN WAVES ☐   PAIN FLARE ☐

WORSE IN MORNING ☐

Notes

_____

_____

_____

_____

_____

_____

_____

_____

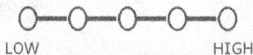

Today's Water Intake

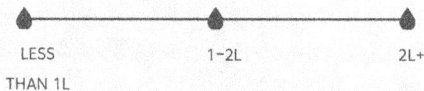

LESS THAN 1L   1-2L   2L+

Food & Immune Response

DID YOU EAT ANYTHING NEW TODAY?

YES ☐   NO ☐

Impact On Symptoms

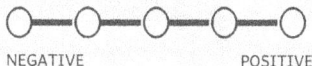

O—O—O—O—O

NEGATIVE   POSITIVE

Notes

_____

_____

_____

_____

_____

_____

Activity Overview

REST DAY ☐   LIGHT MOVEMENT ☐

MODERATE ACTIVITY ☐   HEAVY ACTIVITY ☐

Effect On Pain   WORSE O—O—O—O—O BETTER

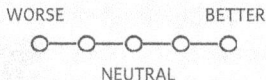

NEUTRAL

DAILY SYMPTOM TRACKER

Date:

Sleep	
QUALITY (1-10) _____	LENGTH _____

Flare Status
SUDDEN ☐ TRIGGERED ☐
SLOW BUILDING ☐ RANDOM ☐

NO FLARE ○ ○ ○ ○ ○ SEVERE FLAIR
MILD   MODERATE

Weather
HOT ☐ DRY ☐ HUMID ☐
RAIN ☐ STORM ☐ COLD ☐

SUSPECTED TRIGGER _____

Today's Symptoms

	LOW	HIGH
FEVER	○—○—○—○—○	
FATIGUE	○—○—○—○—○	

Systemic

DIZZINESS	☐	NIGHT SWEATS	☐
WEIGHT CHANGE	☐	FLUE-LIKE	☐
CHILLS	☐	BRAIN FOG	☐

Pain & Inflammation

JOINT PAIN	☐	JOINT SWELLING	☐
STIFFNESS	☐	MUSCLE ACHES	☐
WEAKNESS	☐	BACK PAIN	☐
NERVE PAIN	☐	MIGRAINES	☐

Thyroid-like

TREMORS	☐	HEART PALPITATIONS	☐
HEAT/COLD SENSITITVITY	☐	WEIGHT SHIFT	☐
CHILLS	☐	NECK PAIN	☐

Skin, Hair & Nails

RASH	☐	REDNESS/FLUSHING	☐
HIVES	☐	SENSITITY TO SUN	☐
ITCHING	☐	BRITTLE NAILS	☐
HAIR LOSS	☐	DRY SKIN	☐

Respiratory

CHEST PAIN	☐	CHRONIC COUGH	☐
SHORTNESS OF BREATH	☐		

Kidneys

FOAMY URINE	☐	SWELLING IN LEGS / ANKLES	☐
DARK URINE	☐	BLOODY URINE	☐

Digestive / GI

NAUSEA	☐	STOMACH PAINS	☐
VOMITING	☐	FOOD REACTIONS	☐
DIARRHEA	☐	APPETITE LOSS	☐
CONSTIPATION	☐	BLOATING	☐

Vascular

NUMB FINGERS/TOES	☐	RAYNAUD'S COLOR CHANGES	☐

DAILY SYMPTOM TRACKER

Date:

Stress Level O—O—O—O—O
 LOW   HIGH

Pain's Impact On Today's Function
Today pain affected my ability to:

DRIVE ☐   WORK ☐   SOCIALIZE ☐

COOK ☐   LIFT/CARRY ☐   LEAVE THE ☐
                         HOUSE

WALK ☐   CARE FOR ☐   SIT/LAY ☐
          SELF   DOWN

Symptom Changes Throughout The Day

CONSISTENT ☐   WORSE AT NIGHT ☐

COMES IN WAVES ☐   PAIN FLARE ☐

WORSE IN MORNING ☐

Notes

_____

_____

_____

_____

_____

_____

_____

_____

Today's Water Intake

LESS   1–2L   2L+
THAN 1L

Food & Immune Response
DID YOU EAT ANYTHING NEW TODAY?
  YES ☐   NO ☐

Impact On Symptoms

O—O—O—O—O
NEGATIVE   POSITIVE

Notes

_____

_____

_____

_____

_____

_____

_____

Activity Overview

REST DAY ☐   LIGHT MOVEMENT ☐

MODERATE ACTIVITY ☐   HEAVY ACTIVITY ☐

              WORSE   BETTER
Effect On Pain   O—O—O—O—O
              NEUTRAL

DAILY SYMPTOM TRACKER

Date:

Sleep QUALITY (1-10) _____ LENGTH _____

Flare Status
SUDDEN ☐ TRIGGERED ☐
SLOW BUILDING ☐ RANDOM ☐

NO FLARE ○ ○ ○ ○ ○ SEVERE FLAIR
MILD   MODERATE

Weather
HOT ☐ DRY ☐ HUMID ☐
RAIN ☐ STORM ☐ COLD ☐

SUSPECTED TRIGGER _____

Today's Symptoms

	LOW	HIGH
FEVER	○—○—○—○—○	
FATIGUE	○—○—○—○—○	

Pain & Inflammation

JOINT PAIN ☐   JOINT SWELLING ☐

STIFFNESS ☐   MUSCLE ACHES ☐

WEAKNESS ☐   BACK PAIN ☐

NERVE PAIN ☐   MIGRAINES ☐

Skin, Hair & Nails

RASH ☐   REDNESS/FLUSHING ☐

HIVES ☐   SENSITITY TO SUN ☐

ITCHING ☐   BRITTLE NAILS ☐

HAIR LOSS ☐   DRY SKIN ☐

Digestive / GI

NAUSEA ☐   STOMACH PAINS ☐

VOMITING ☐   FOOD REACTIONS ☐

DIARRHEA ☐   APPETITE LOSS ☐

CONSTIPATION ☐   BLOATING ☐

Systemic

DIZZINESS ☐   NIGHT SWEATS ☐

WEIGHT CHANGE ☐   FLUE-LIKE ☐

CHILLS ☐   BRAIN FOG ☐

Thyroid-like

TREMORS ☐   HEART PALPITATIONS ☐

HEAT/COLD SENSITITVITY ☐   WEIGHT SHIFT ☐

CHILLS ☐   NECK PAIN ☐

Respiratory

CHEST PAIN ☐   CHRONIC COUGH ☐

SHORTNESS OF BREATH ☐

Kidneys

FOAMY URINE ☐   SWELLING IN LEGS / ANKLES ☐

DARK URINE ☐   BLOODY URINE ☐

Vascular

NUMB FINGERS/TOES ☐   RAYNAUD'S COLOR CHANGES ☐

DAILY SYMPTOM TRACKER

Date:

Stress Level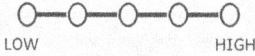
LOW   HIGH

Pain's Impact On Today's Function
Today pain affected my ability to:

DRIVE ☐   WORK ☐   SOCIALIZE ☐

COOK ☐   LIFT/CARRY ☐   LEAVE THE HOUSE ☐

WALK ☐   CARE FOR SELF ☐   SIT/LAY DOWN ☐

Symptom Changes Throughout The Day

CONSISTENT ☐   WORSE AT NIGHT ☐

COMES IN WAVES ☐   PAIN FLARE ☐

WORSE IN MORNING ☐

Notes

_____

_____

_____

_____

_____

_____

_____

_____

Today's Water Intake

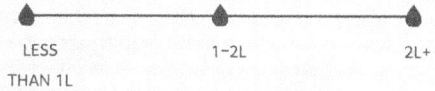

LESS THAN 1L   1–2L   2L+

Food & Immune Response

DID YOU EAT ANYTHING NEW TODAY?

YES ☐   NO ☐

Impact On Symptoms

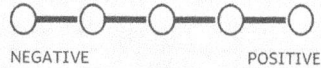

NEGATIVE   POSITIVE

Notes

_____

_____

_____

_____

_____

_____

Activity Overview

REST DAY ☐   LIGHT MOVEMENT ☐

MODERATE ACTIVITY ☐   HEAVY ACTIVITY ☐

WORSE   BETTER

Effect On Pain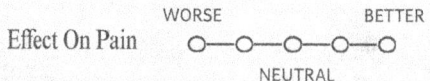

NEUTRAL

IMPORTANT NOTES

WEEKLY SUMMARY

Week Of:

Sleep	Overall Feelings
QUALITY (1–10) _____	MOOD (1–10) _____ MENTAL CLARITY (1–10) _____ ENERGY (1–10) _____ IMPACT FROM WEATHER (1–10) _____

Autoimmune Flare Snapshot

This week:

I EXPERIENCED UNUSUAL FATIGUE	NOT AT ALL ☐	SEVERAL TIMES ☐	OFTEN ☐	CONSTANT ☐
MY PAIN WAS	LOW ☐	MILD ☐	WORSE ☐	CONSTANT ☐
I HAD MORNING STIFFNESS	NOT AT ALL ☐	30 MINUTES ☐	30-60 ☐	OVER 60 ☐
MY SYMPTOMS WORSENED WITH ACTIVITY	NOT AT ALL ☐	SEVERAL TIMES ☐	OFTEN ☐	CONSTANT ☐
MY SYMPTOMS WORSENED WITH REST	NOT AT ALL ☐	SEVERAL TIMES ☐	OFTEN ☐	CONSTANT ☐
I HAD FLU-LIKE SENSATIONS	NOT AT ALL ☐	SEVERAL TIMES ☐	OFTEN ☐	CONSTANT ☐

FATIGUE & ENERGY CHECK-IN

This week made feel:

FEELING "POISONED" OR SICK	NOT AT ALL ☐	SEVERAL TIMES ☐	OFTEN ☐	CONSTANT ☐
EXHAUSTION AFTER SMALL TASKS	NOT AT ALL ☐	SEVERAL TIMES ☐	OFTEN ☐	CONSTANT ☐
FEELING TIRED EVEN AFTER RESTING	NOT AT ALL ☐	SEVERAL TIMES ☐	OFTEN ☐	CONSTANT ☐
MUSCLES FEELING WEAK OR "HEAVY"	NOT AT ALL ☐	SEVERAL TIMES ☐	OFTEN ☐	CONSTANT ☐
NEEDING NAPS TO FUNCTION	NOT AT ALL ☐	SEVERAL TIMES ☐	OFTEN ☐	CONSTANT ☐
BRAIN FOG INTERFERING WITH THINKING	NOT AT ALL ☐	SEVERAL TIMES ☐	OFTEN ☐	CONSTANT ☐

MOBILITY CHECK-IN

During this week, how often did you experience:

STIFFNESS IN THE MORNING	NOT AT ALL ☐	SEVERAL TIMES ☐	OFTEN ☐	CONSTANT ☐
DIFFICULTY GETTING OUT OF BED	NOT AT ALL ☐	SEVERAL TIMES ☐	OFTEN ☐	CONSTANT ☐
REDUCED RANGE OF MOTION	NOT AT ALL ☐	SEVERAL TIMES ☐	OFTEN ☐	CONSTANT ☐
TROUBLE GRIPPING OR LIFTING	NOT AT ALL ☐	SEVERAL TIMES ☐	OFTEN ☐	CONSTANT ☐
SLOWER WALKING SPEED	NOT AT ALL ☐	SEVERAL TIMES ☐	OFTEN ☐	CONSTANT ☐
FEELING UNSTABLE OR WEAK	NOT AT ALL ☐	SEVERAL TIMES ☐	OFTEN ☐	CONSTANT ☐
NEEDED MOBILITY AIDS	NOT AT ALL ☐	SEVERAL TIMES ☐	OFTEN ☐	CONSTANT ☐

WEEKLY SUMMARY

Week Of:

Sleep

QUALITY (1-10) _____

Overall Feelings

MOOD (1-10) _____ MENTAL CLARITY (1-10) _____

ENERGY (1-10) _____ IMPACT FROM WEATHER (1-10) _____

RED FLAG CHECK-IN

During this week, did you notice:

NEW NUMBNESS	NOT AT ALL ☐	SEVERAL TIMES ☐	OFTEN ☐	CONSTANT ☐
NEW WEAKNESS	NOT AT ALL ☐	SEVERAL TIMES ☐	OFTEN ☐	CONSTANT ☐
PAIN THAT WOKE ME FROM SLEEP	NOT AT ALL ☐	SEVERAL TIMES ☐	OFTEN ☐	CONSTANT ☐
LOSS OF BLADDER/BOWEL CONTROL	NOT AT ALL ☐	SEVERAL TIMES ☐	OFTEN ☐	CONSTANT ☐
SUDDEN SEVERE PAIN	NOT AT ALL ☐	SEVERAL TIMES ☐	OFTEN ☐	CONSTANT ☐
NEW SWELLING/REDNESS	NOT AT ALL ☐	SEVERAL TIMES ☐	OFTEN ☐	CONSTANT ☐

IT IS ESSENTIAL TO BRING THESE RESULTS UP WITH YOUR HEALTHCARE PROVIDER AS SOON AS POSSIBLE.

FLARE PATTERN CHECK-IN

During this week, I had flares that felt:

SUDDEN	NOT AT ALL ☐	SEVERAL TIMES ☐	OFTEN ☐
SLOW-BUILDING	NOT AT ALL ☐	SEVERAL TIMES ☐	OFTEN ☐
TRIGGERED	NOT AT ALL ☐	SEVERAL TIMES ☐	OFTEN ☐
RANDOM	NOT AT ALL ☐	SEVERAL TIMES ☐	OFTEN ☐
WORSE THAN USUAL	NOT AT ALL ☐	SEVERAL TIMES ☐	OFTEN ☐
UNUSUAL COMPARED TO TYPICAL FLARES	NOT AT ALL ☐	SEVERAL TIMES ☐	OFTEN ☐

DURATION OF FLARES _____

Notes

_____

_____

_____

_____

WEEKLY SUMMARY
PATTERNS & NOTES

Week Of:

Patterns / Similarities On Good Days

- ○ _____
- ○ _____
- ○ _____
- ○ _____
- ○ _____

Patterns / Similarities On Bad Days

- ○ _____
- ○ _____
- ○ _____
- ○ _____
- ○ _____

Things That Improved Symptoms

- ○ _____
- ○ _____
- ○ _____
- ○ _____
- ○ _____

WEEKLY SUMMARY
PATTERNS & NOTES

Week Of:

Most Common Symptoms

○ _____
○ _____
○ _____
○ _____
○ _____

Most Common Triggers

○ _____
○ _____
○ _____
○ _____
○ _____

Symptom Timing Patterns

When do your symptoms tend to be at their worst?

MORNING ☐   AFTER MEALS ☐
AFTERNOON ☐   AFTER PHYSICAL ACTIVITY ☐
EVENING ☐   HORMONE FLUCTUATIONS ☐
NIGHT ☐   DURING STRESS ☐
UPON WAKING ☐   DURING WEATHER CHANGES ☐

Overall Effectiveness Of Treatment This Week

○———○———○———○———○
LOW   HIGH

Overall Stress This Week

○———○———○———○———○
LOW   HIGH

Overall Sleep This Week

○———○———○———○———○
LOW   HIGH

NOTES

_____
_____
_____
_____
_____
_____
_____
_____
_____
_____
_____
_____
_____
_____
_____
_____

IMPORTANT NOTES

NEW WEEK CHECK-IN
PATTERNS & NOTES

How Did Last Week Go Overall?   O———O———O———O———O

MUCH WORSE   MUCH BETTER

Any Clear Patterns Or Triggers?   New Things You're Trying This Week

O _____   O _____
O _____   O _____
O _____   O _____
O _____   O _____
O _____   O _____

Changes To Medication/Supplements?   YES ☐   NO ☐

NOTE: _____

Changes To Treatment/Therapies?   YES ☐   NO ☐

NOTE: _____

Emotional & Mental Health Check-In

HOW ARE YOU FEELING HEADING INTO THIS WEEK? ANYTHING WEIGHING ON YOU?

_____
_____
_____
_____
_____
_____
_____

DAILY SYMPTOM TRACKER

Date:

Sleep QUALITY (1-10) _____ LENGTH _____

Weather
HOT ☐ DRY ☐ HUMID ☐
RAIN ☐ STORM ☐ COLD ☐

Flare Status
SUDDEN ☐ TRIGGERED ☐
SLOW BUILDING ☐ RANDOM ☐

NO FLARE ○ ○ ○ ○ ○ SEVERE FLAIR
MILD   MODERATE

SUSPECTED TRIGGER _____

Today's Symptoms

Systemic

	LOW	HIGH
FEVER	○—○—○—○—○	
FATIGUE	○—○—○—○—○	

DIZZINESS ☐   NIGHT SWEATS ☐
WEIGHT CHANGE ☐   FLUE-LIKE ☐
CHILLS ☐   BRAIN FOG ☐

Pain & Inflammation

JOINT PAIN ☐   JOINT SWELLING ☐
STIFFNESS ☐   MUSCLE ACHES ☐
WEAKNESS ☐   BACK PAIN ☐
NERVE PAIN ☐   MIGRAINES ☐

Thyroid-like

TREMORS ☐   HEART PALPITATIONS ☐
HEAT/COLD SENSITITVITY ☐   WEIGHT SHIFT ☐
CHILLS ☐   NECK PAIN ☐

Skin, Hair & Nails

RASH ☐   REDNESS/FLUSHING ☐
HIVES ☐   SENSITITITY TO SUN ☐
ITCHING ☐   BRITTLE NAILS ☐
HAIR LOSS ☐   DRY SKIN ☐

Respiratory

CHEST PAIN ☐   CHRONIC COUGH ☐
SHORTNESS OF BREATH ☐

Kidneys

FOAMY URINE ☐   SWELLING IN LEGS / ANKLES ☐
DARK URINE ☐   BLOODY URINE ☐

Digestive / GI

NAUSEA ☐   STOMACH PAINS ☐
VOMITING ☐   FOOD REACTIONS ☐
DIARRHEA ☐   APPETITE LOSS ☐
CONSTIPATION ☐   BLOATING ☐

Vascular

NUMB FINGERS/TOES ☐   RAYNAUD'S COLOR CHANGES ☐

DAILY SYMPTOM TRACKER

Date:

Stress Level

O—O—O—O—O

LOW   HIGH

Pain's Impact On Today's Function
Today pain affected my ability to:

DRIVE ☐   WORK ☐   SOCIALIZE ☐

COOK ☐   LIFT/CARRY ☐   LEAVE THE HOUSE ☐

WALK ☐   CARE FOR SELF ☐   SIT/LAY DOWN ☐

Symptom Changes Throughout The Day

CONSISTENT ☐   WORSE AT NIGHT ☐

COMES IN WAVES ☐   PAIN FLARE ☐

WORSE IN MORNING ☐

Notes

_____

_____

_____

_____

_____

_____

_____

_____

_____

Today's Water Intake

◆————◆————◆

LESS THAN 1L   1–2L   2L+

Food & Immune Response

DID YOU EAT ANYTHING NEW TODAY?

YES ☐   NO ☐

Impact On Symptoms

O—O—O—O—O

NEGATIVE   POSITIVE

Notes

_____

_____

_____

_____

_____

_____

Activity Overview

REST DAY ☐   LIGHT MOVEMENT ☐

MODERATE ACTIVITY ☐   HEAVY ACTIVITY ☐

Effect On Pain   O—O—O—O—O

        WORSE   BETTER

            NEUTRAL

DAILY SYMPTOM TRACKER

Date:

Sleep QUALITY (1-10) _____ LENGTH _____

Weather
HOT ☐ DRY ☐ HUMID ☐
RAIN ☐ STORM ☐ COLD ☐

Flare Status
SUDDEN ☐ TRIGGERED ☐
SLOW BUILDING ☐ RANDOM ☐

NO FLARE ○ ○ ○ ○ ○ SEVERE FLAIR
MILD MODERATE

SUSPECTED TRIGGER _____

Today's Symptoms

	LOW	HIGH
FEVER	○—○—○—○—○	
FATIGUE	○—○—○—○—○	

Systemic

DIZZINESS ☐ NIGHT SWEATS ☐
WEIGHT CHANGE ☐ FLUE–LIKE ☐
CHILLS ☐ BRAIN FOG ☐

Pain & Inflammation

JOINT PAIN ☐ JOINT SWELLING ☐
STIFFNESS ☐ MUSCLE ACHES ☐
WEAKNESS ☐ BACK PAIN ☐
NERVE PAIN ☐ MIGRAINES ☐

Thyroid-like

TREMORS ☐ HEART PALPITATIONS ☐
HEAT/COLD SENSITITVITY ☐ WEIGHT SHIFT ☐
CHILLS ☐ NECK PAIN ☐

Skin, Hair & Nails

RASH ☐ REDNESS/FLUSHING ☐
HIVES ☐ SENSITITITY TO SUN ☐
ITCHING ☐ BRITTLE NAILS ☐
HAIR LOSS ☐ DRY SKIN ☐

Respiratory

CHEST PAIN ☐ CHRONIC COUGH ☐
SHORTNESS OF BREATH ☐

Kidneys

FOAMY URINE ☐ SWELLING IN LEGS / ANKLES ☐
DARK URINE ☐ BLOODY URINE ☐

Digestive / GI

NAUSEA ☐ STOMACH PAINS ☐
VOMITING ☐ FOOD REACTIONS ☐
DIARRHEA ☐ APPETITE LOSS ☐
CONSTIPATION ☐ BLOATING ☐

Vascular

NUMB FINGERS/TOES ☐ RAYNAUD'S COLOR CHANGES ☐

DAILY SYMPTOM TRACKER

Date:

Stress Level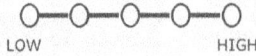
LOW   HIGH

Pain's Impact On Today's Function
Today pain affected my ability to:

DRIVE ☐   WORK ☐   SOCIALIZE ☐

COOK ☐   LIFT/CARRY ☐   LEAVE THE HOUSE ☐

WALK ☐   CARE FOR SELF ☐   SIT/LAY DOWN ☐

Symptom Changes Throughout The Day

CONSISTENT ☐   WORSE AT NIGHT ☐

COMES IN WAVES ☐   PAIN FLARE ☐

WORSE IN MORNING ☐

Notes

_____

_____

_____

_____

_____

_____

_____

_____

_____

Today's Water Intake

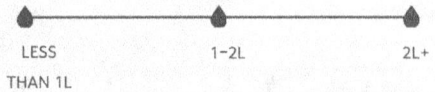
LESS THAN 1L   1–2L   2L+

Food & Immune Response
DID YOU EAT ANYTHING NEW TODAY?

YES ☐   NO ☐

Impact On Symptoms

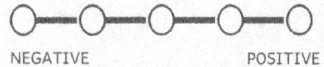
NEGATIVE   POSITIVE

Notes

_____

_____

_____

_____

_____

_____

_____

Activity Overview

REST DAY ☐   LIGHT MOVEMENT ☐

MODERATE ACTIVITY ☐   HEAVY ACTIVITY ☐

WORSE   BETTER

Effect On Pain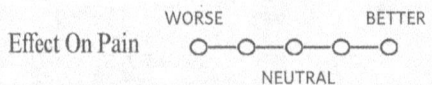
NEUTRAL

DAILY SYMPTOM TRACKER

Date:

Sleep QUALITY (1-10) _____ LENGTH _____

Flare Status
SUDDEN ☐ TRIGGERED ☐
SLOW BUILDING ☐ RANDOM ☐

NO FLARE ○ ○ ○ ○ ○ SEVERE FLAIR
  MILD   MODERATE

SUSPECTED TRIGGER _____

Weather
HOT ☐ DRY ☐ HUMID ☐
RAIN ☐ STORM ☐ COLD ☐

Today's Symptoms

	LOW	HIGH
FEVER	○—○—○—○—○	
FATIGUE	○—○—○—○—○	

Pain & Inflammation

JOINT PAIN ☐	JOINT SWELLING ☐
STIFFNESS ☐	MUSCLE ACHES ☐
WEAKNESS ☐	BACK PAIN ☐
NERVE PAIN ☐	MIGRAINES ☐

Skin, Hair & Nails

RASH ☐	REDNESS/FLUSHING ☐
HIVES ☐	SENSITITITY TO SUN ☐
ITCHING ☐	BRITTLE NAILS ☐
HAIR LOSS ☐	DRY SKIN ☐

Digestive / GI

NAUSEA ☐	STOMACH PAINS ☐
VOMITING ☐	FOOD REACTIONS ☐
DIARRHEA ☐	APPETITE LOSS ☐
CONSTIPATION ☐	BLOATING ☐

Systemic

DIZZINESS ☐	NIGHT SWEATS ☐
WEIGHT CHANGE ☐	FLUE-LIKE ☐
CHILLS ☐	BRAIN FOG ☐

Thyroid-like

TREMORS ☐	HEART PALPITATIONS ☐
HEAT/COLD SENSITITVITY ☐	WEIGHT SHIFT ☐
CHILLS ☐	NECK PAIN ☐

Respiratory

CHEST PAIN ☐	CHRONIC COUGH ☐
SHORTNESS OF BREATH ☐	

Kidneys

FOAMY URINE ☐	SWELLING IN LEGS / ANKLES ☐
DARK URINE ☐	BLOODY URINE ☐

Vascular

NUMB FINGERS/TOES ☐	RAYNAUD'S COLOR CHANGES ☐

DAILY SYMPTOM TRACKER

Date:

Stress Level

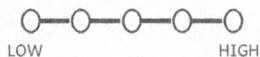

LOW   HIGH

Pain's Impact On Today's Function
Today pain affected my ability to:

DRIVE ☐   WORK ☐   SOCIALIZE ☐

COOK ☐   LIFT/CARRY ☐   LEAVE THE HOUSE ☐

WALK ☐   CARE FOR SELF ☐   SIT/LAY DOWN ☐

Symptom Changes Throughout The Day

CONSISTENT ☐   WORSE AT NIGHT ☐

COMES IN WAVES ☐   PAIN FLARE ☐

WORSE IN MORNING ☐

Notes

_____

_____

_____

_____

_____

_____

_____

_____

_____

Today's Water Intake

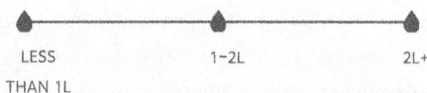

LESS THAN 1L   1–2L   2L+

Food & Immune Response

DID YOU EAT ANYTHING NEW TODAY?

YES ☐   NO ☐

Impact On Symptoms

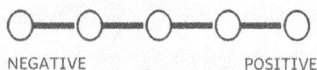

NEGATIVE   POSITIVE

Notes

_____

_____

_____

_____

_____

_____

Activity Overview

REST DAY ☐   LIGHT MOVEMENT ☐

MODERATE ACTIVITY ☐   HEAVY ACTIVITY ☐

Effect On Pain

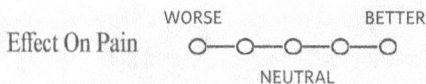

WORSE   BETTER

NEUTRAL

DAILY SYMPTOM TRACKER

Date:

Sleep QUALITY (1-10) _____ LENGTH _____

Flare Status
SUDDEN ☐ TRIGGERED ☐
SLOW BUILDING ☐ RANDOM ☐

NO FLARE ○ ○ ○ ○ ○ SEVERE FLAIR
MILD   MODERATE

SUSPECTED TRIGGER _____

Weather
HOT ☐ DRY ☐ HUMID ☐
RAIN ☐ STORM ☐ COLD ☐

Today's Symptoms

	LOW	HIGH
FEVER	○—○—○—○—○	
FATIGUE	○—○—○—○—○	

Systemic

DIZZINESS	☐	NIGHT SWEATS	☐
WEIGHT CHANGE	☐	FLUE-LIKE	☐
CHILLS	☐	BRAIN FOG	☐

Pain & Inflammation

JOINT PAIN	☐	JOINT SWELLING	☐
STIFFNESS	☐	MUSCLE ACHES	☐
WEAKNESS	☐	BACK PAIN	☐
NERVE PAIN	☐	MIGRAINES	☐

Thyroid-like

TREMORS	☐	HEART PALPITATIONS	☐
HEAT/COLD SENSITITVITY	☐	WEIGHT SHIFT	☐
CHILLS	☐	NECK PAIN	☐

Skin, Hair & Nails

RASH	☐	REDNESS/FLUSHING	☐
HIVES	☐	SENSITITY TO SUN	☐
ITCHING	☐	BRITTLE NAILS	☐
HAIR LOSS	☐	DRY SKIN	☐

Respiratory

CHEST PAIN	☐	CHRONIC COUGH	☐
SHORTNESS OF BREATH	☐		

Kidneys

FOAMY URINE	☐	SWELLING IN LEGS / ANKLES	☐
DARK URINE	☐	BLOODY URINE	☐

Digestive / GI

NAUSEA	☐	STOMACH PAINS	☐
VOMITING	☐	FOOD REACTIONS	☐
DIARRHEA	☐	APPETITE LOSS	☐
CONSTIPATION	☐	BLOATING	☐

Vascular

NUMB FINGERS/TOES	☐	RAYNAUD'S COLOR CHANGES	☐

DAILY SYMPTOM TRACKER

Date:

Stress Level

O—O—O—O—O
LOW   HIGH

Pain's Impact On Today's Function
Today pain affected my ability to:

DRIVE ☐   WORK ☐   SOCIALIZE ☐

COOK ☐   LIFT/CARRY ☐   LEAVE THE HOUSE ☐

WALK ☐   CARE FOR SELF ☐   SIT/LAY DOWN ☐

Symptom Changes Throughout The Day

CONSISTENT ☐   WORSE AT NIGHT ☐

COMES IN WAVES ☐   PAIN FLARE ☐

WORSE IN MORNING ☐

Notes

_____

_____

_____

_____

_____

_____

_____

_____

Today's Water Intake

LESS THAN 1L   1–2L   2L+

Food & Immune Response

DID YOU EAT ANYTHING NEW TODAY?

YES ☐   NO ☐

Impact On Symptoms

O—O—O—O—O
NEGATIVE   POSITIVE

Notes

_____

_____

_____

_____

_____

_____

Activity Overview

REST DAY ☐   LIGHT MOVEMENT ☐

MODERATE ACTIVITY ☐   HEAVY ACTIVITY ☐

Effect On Pain   WORSE   BETTER

O—O—O—O—O

NEUTRAL

DAILY SYMPTOM TRACKER

Date:

Sleep
QUALITY (1-10) _____ LENGTH _____

Flare Status
SUDDEN ☐ TRIGGERED ☐
SLOW BUILDING ☐ RANDOM ☐

NO FLARE ○ ○ ○ ○ ○ SEVERE FLAIR
MILD MODERATE

SUSPECTED TRIGGER _____

Weather
HOT ☐ DRY ☐ HUMID ☐
RAIN ☐ STORM ☐ COLD ☐

Today's Symptoms

	LOW				HIGH
FEVER	○—○—○—○—○
FATIGUE	○—○—○—○—○

Systemic

DIZZINESS	☐	NIGHT SWEATS	☐
WEIGHT CHANGE	☐	FLUE-LIKE	☐
CHILLS	☐	BRAIN FOG	☐

Pain & Inflammation

JOINT PAIN	☐	JOINT SWELLING	☐
STIFFNESS	☐	MUSCLE ACHES	☐
WEAKNESS	☐	BACK PAIN	☐
NERVE PAIN	☐	MIGRAINES	☐

Thyroid-like

TREMORS	☐	HEART PALPITATIONS	☐
HEAT/COLD SENSITITVITY	☐	WEIGHT SHIFT	☐
CHILLS	☐	NECK PAIN	☐

Skin, Hair & Nails

RASH	☐	REDNESS/FLUSHING	☐
HIVES	☐	SENSITITY TO SUN	☐
ITCHING	☐	BRITTLE NAILS	☐
HAIR LOSS	☐	DRY SKIN	☐

Respiratory

CHEST PAIN	☐	CHRONIC COUGH	☐
SHORTNESS OF BREATH	☐		

Kidneys

FOAMY URINE	☐	SWELLING IN LEGS / ANKLES	☐
DARK URINE	☐	BLOODY URINE	☐

Digestive / GI

NAUSEA	☐	STOMACH PAINS	☐
VOMITING	☐	FOOD REACTIONS	☐
DIARRHEA	☐	APPETITE LOSS	☐
CONSTIPATION	☐	BLOATING	☐

Vascular

NUMB FINGERS/TOES	☐	RAYNAUD'S COLOR CHANGES	☐

DAILY SYMPTOM TRACKER

Date:

Stress Level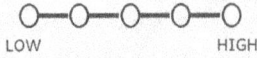
LOW   HIGH

Pain's Impact On Today's Function
Today pain affected my ability to:

DRIVE ☐   WORK ☐   SOCIALIZE ☐

COOK ☐   LIFT/CARRY ☐   LEAVE THE HOUSE ☐

WALK ☐   CARE FOR SELF ☐   SIT/LAY DOWN ☐

Symptom Changes Throughout The Day

CONSISTENT ☐   WORSE AT NIGHT ☐

COMES IN WAVES ☐   PAIN FLARE ☐

WORSE IN MORNING ☐

Notes

_____

_____

_____

_____

_____

_____

_____

_____

_____

Today's Water Intake

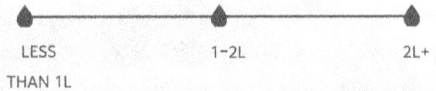
LESS THAN 1L   1-2L   2L+

Food & Immune Response
DID YOU EAT ANYTHING NEW TODAY?
YES ☐   NO ☐

Impact On Symptoms

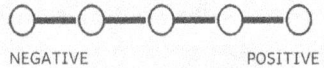
NEGATIVE   POSITIVE

Notes

_____

_____

_____

_____

_____

_____

Activity Overview

REST DAY ☐   LIGHT MOVEMENT ☐

MODERATE ACTIVITY ☐   HEAVY ACTIVITY ☐

WORSE   BETTER

Effect On Pain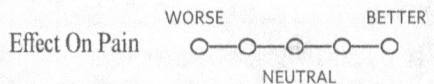
NEUTRAL

DAILY SYMPTOM TRACKER

Date:

Sleep QUALITY (1-10) _____ LENGTH _____

Flare Status
SUDDEN ☐ TRIGGERED ☐
SLOW BUILDING ☐ RANDOM ☐

NO FLARE ○ ○ ○ ○ ○ SEVERE FLAIR
MILD   MODERATE

SUSPECTED TRIGGER _____

Weather
HOT ☐ DRY ☐ HUMID ☐
RAIN ☐ STORM ☐ COLD ☐

Today's Symptoms

LOW   HIGH

FEVER   ○—○—○—○—○
FATIGUE   ○—○—○—○—○

Systemic

DIZZINESS ☐   NIGHT SWEATS ☐
WEIGHT CHANGE ☐   FLUE-LIKE ☐
CHILLS ☐   BRAIN FOG ☐

Pain & Inflammation

JOINT PAIN ☐   JOINT SWELLING ☐
STIFFNESS ☐   MUSCLE ACHES ☐
WEAKNESS ☐   BACK PAIN ☐
NERVE PAIN ☐   MIGRAINES ☐

Thyroid-like

TREMORS ☐   HEART PALPITATIONS ☐
HEAT/COLD SENSITITVITY ☐   WEIGHT SHIFT ☐
CHILLS ☐   NECK PAIN ☐

Skin, Hair & Nails

RASH ☐   REDNESS/FLUSHING ☐
HIVES ☐   SENSITITY TO SUN ☐
ITCHING ☐   BRITTLE NAILS ☐
HAIR LOSS ☐   DRY SKIN ☐

Respiratory

CHEST PAIN ☐   CHRONIC COUGH ☐
SHORTNESS OF BREATH ☐

Kidneys

FOAMY URINE ☐   SWELLING IN LEGS / ANKLES ☐
DARK URINE ☐   BLOODY URINE ☐

Digestive / GI

NAUSEA ☐   STOMACH PAINS ☐
VOMITING ☐   FOOD REACTIONS ☐
DIARRHEA ☐   APPETITE LOSS ☐
CONSTIPATION ☐   BLOATING ☐

Vascular

NUMB FINGERS/TOES ☐   RAYNAUD'S COLOR CHANGES ☐

DAILY SYMPTOM TRACKER

Date: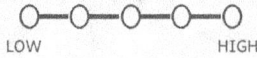

Stress Level

O—O—O—O—O

LOW   HIGH

Today's Water Intake

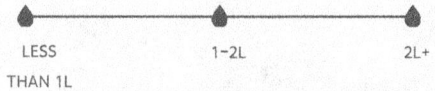

LESS THAN 1L   1–2L   2L+

Pain's Impact On Today's Function

Today pain affected my ability to:

DRIVE ☐	WORK ☐	SOCIALIZE ☐
COOK ☐	LIFT/CARRY ☐	LEAVE THE HOUSE ☐
WALK ☐	CARE FOR SELF ☐	SIT/LAY DOWN ☐

Food & Immune Response

DID YOU EAT ANYTHING NEW TODAY?

YES ☐   NO ☐

Impact On Symptoms

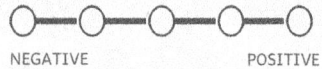

NEGATIVE   POSITIVE

Notes

_____
_____
_____
_____
_____
_____
_____

Symptom Changes Throughout The Day

CONSISTENT ☐	WORSE AT NIGHT ☐
COMES IN WAVES ☐	PAIN FLARE ☐
WORSE IN MORNING ☐	

Notes

_____
_____
_____
_____
_____
_____
_____
_____
_____

Activity Overview

REST DAY ☐	LIGHT MOVEMENT ☐
MODERATE ACTIVITY ☐	HEAVY ACTIVITY ☐

Effect On Pain

WORSE   BETTER

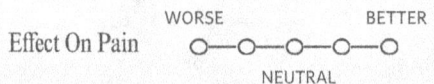

NEUTRAL

DAILY SYMPTOM TRACKER

Date:

Sleep QUALITY (1-10) _____ LENGTH _____

Flare Status
SUDDEN ☐ TRIGGERED ☐
SLOW BUILDING ☐ RANDOM ☐

NO FLARE ○ ○ ○ ○ ○ SEVERE FLAIR
MILD   MODERATE

Weather
HOT ☐ DRY ☐ HUMID ☐
RAIN ☐ STORM ☐ COLD ☐

SUSPECTED TRIGGER _____

Today's Symptoms

	LOW	HIGH
FEVER	○—○—○—○—○	
FATIGUE	○—○—○—○—○	

Systemic

DIZZINESS	☐	NIGHT SWEATS	☐
WEIGHT CHANGE	☐	FLUE-LIKE	☐
CHILLS	☐	BRAIN FOG	☐

Pain & Inflammation

JOINT PAIN	☐	JOINT SWELLING	☐
STIFFNESS	☐	MUSCLE ACHES	☐
WEAKNESS	☐	BACK PAIN	☐
NERVE PAIN	☐	MIGRAINES	☐

Thyroid-like

TREMORS	☐	HEART PALPITATIONS	☐
HEAT/COLD SENSITITVITY	☐	WEIGHT SHIFT	☐
CHILLS	☐	NECK PAIN	☐

Skin, Hair & Nails

RASH	☐	REDNESS/FLUSHING	☐
HIVES	☐	SENSITITY TO SUN	☐
ITCHING	☐	BRITTLE NAILS	☐
HAIR LOSS	☐	DRY SKIN	☐

Respiratory

CHEST PAIN	☐	CHRONIC COUGH	☐
SHORTNESS OF BREATH	☐		

Kidneys

FOAMY URINE	☐	SWELLING IN LEGS / ANKLES	☐
DARK URINE	☐	BLOODY URINE	☐

Digestive / GI

NAUSEA	☐	STOMACH PAINS	☐
VOMITING	☐	FOOD REACTIONS	☐
DIARRHEA	☐	APPETITE LOSS	☐
CONSTIPATION	☐	BLOATING	☐

Vascular

NUMB FINGERS/TOES	☐	RAYNAUD'S COLOR CHANGES	☐

DAILY SYMPTOM TRACKER

Date:

Stress Level

O—O—O—O—O

LOW   HIGH

Pain's Impact On Today's Function
Today pain affected my ability to:

DRIVE ☐   WORK ☐   SOCIALIZE ☐

COOK ☐   LIFT/CARRY ☐   LEAVE THE HOUSE ☐

WALK ☐   CARE FOR SELF ☐   SIT/LAY DOWN ☐

Symptom Changes Throughout The Day

CONSISTENT ☐   WORSE AT NIGHT ☐

COMES IN WAVES ☐   PAIN FLARE ☐

WORSE IN MORNING ☐

Notes

_____

_____

_____

_____

_____

_____

_____

Today's Water Intake

◆———————◆———————◆

LESS THAN 1L   1–2L   2L+

Food & Immune Response

DID YOU EAT ANYTHING NEW TODAY?

YES ☐   NO ☐

Impact On Symptoms

O—O—O—O—O

NEGATIVE   POSITIVE

Notes

_____

_____

_____

_____

_____

_____

Activity Overview

REST DAY ☐   LIGHT MOVEMENT ☐

MODERATE ACTIVITY ☐   HEAVY ACTIVITY ☐

Effect On Pain   O—O—O—O—O

WORSE   NEUTRAL   BETTER

IMPORTANT NOTES

WEEKLY SUMMARY

Week Of:

Sleep	Overall Feelings
QUALITY (1-10) _____	MOOD (1-10) _____ MENTAL CLARITY (1-10) _____
	ENERGY (1-10) _____ IMPACT FROM WEATHER (1-10) _____

Autoimmune Flare Snapshot

This week:

I EXPERIENCED UNUSUAL FATIGUE	NOT AT ALL ☐	SEVERAL TIMES ☐	OFTEN ☐	CONSTANT ☐
MY PAIN WAS	LOW ☐	MILD ☐	WORSE ☐	CONSTANT ☐
I HAD MORNING STIFFNESS	NOT AT ALL ☐	30 MINUTES ☐	30-60 ☐	OVER 60 ☐
MY SYMPTOMS WORSENED WITH ACTIVITY	NOT AT ALL ☐	SEVERAL TIMES ☐	OFTEN ☐	CONSTANT ☐
MY SYMPTOMS WORSENED WITH REST	NOT AT ALL ☐	SEVERAL TIMES ☐	OFTEN ☐	CONSTANT ☐
I HAD FLU-LIKE SENSATIONS	NOT AT ALL ☐	SEVERAL TIMES ☐	OFTEN ☐	CONSTANT ☐

FATIGUE & ENERGY CHECK-IN

This week made feel:

FEELING "POISONED" OR SICK	NOT AT ALL ☐	SEVERAL TIMES ☐	OFTEN ☐	CONSTANT ☐
EXHAUSTION AFTER SMALL TASKS	NOT AT ALL ☐	SEVERAL TIMES ☐	OFTEN ☐	CONSTANT ☐
FEELING TIRED EVEN AFTER RESTING	NOT AT ALL ☐	SEVERAL TIMES ☐	OFTEN ☐	CONSTANT ☐
MUSCLES FEELING WEAK OR "HEAVY"	NOT AT ALL ☐	SEVERAL TIMES ☐	OFTEN ☐	CONSTANT ☐
NEEDING NAPS TO FUNCTION	NOT AT ALL ☐	SEVERAL TIMES ☐	OFTEN ☐	CONSTANT ☐
BRAIN FOG INTERFERING WITH THINKING	NOT AT ALL ☐	SEVERAL TIMES ☐	OFTEN ☐	CONSTANT ☐

MOBILITY CHECK-IN

During this week, how often did you experience:

STIFFNESS IN THE MORNING	NOT AT ALL ☐	SEVERAL TIMES ☐	OFTEN ☐	CONSTANT ☐
DIFFICULTY GETTING OUT OF BED	NOT AT ALL ☐	SEVERAL TIMES ☐	OFTEN ☐	CONSTANT ☐
REDUCED RANGE OF MOTION	NOT AT ALL ☐	SEVERAL TIMES ☐	OFTEN ☐	CONSTANT ☐
TROUBLE GRIPPING OR LIFTING	NOT AT ALL ☐	SEVERAL TIMES ☐	OFTEN ☐	CONSTANT ☐
SLOWER WALKING SPEED	NOT AT ALL ☐	SEVERAL TIMES ☐	OFTEN ☐	CONSTANT ☐
FEELING UNSTABLE OR WEAK	NOT AT ALL ☐	SEVERAL TIMES ☐	OFTEN ☐	CONSTANT ☐
NEEDED MOBILITY AIDS	NOT AT ALL ☐	SEVERAL TIMES ☐	OFTEN ☐	CONSTANT ☐

WEEKLY SUMMARY

Week Of:

Sleep	Overall Feelings
QUALITY (1-10) _____	MOOD (1-10) _____ MENTAL CLARITY (1-10) _____ ENERGY (1-10) _____ IMPACT FROM WEATHER (1-10) _____

RED FLAG CHECK-IN

During this week, did you notice:

NEW NUMBNESS	NOT AT ALL ☐ SEVERAL TIMES ☐	OFTEN ☐	CONSTANT ☐
NEW WEAKNESS	NOT AT ALL ☐ SEVERAL TIMES ☐	OFTEN ☐	CONSTANT ☐
PAIN THAT WOKE ME FROM SLEEP	NOT AT ALL ☐ SEVERAL TIMES ☐	OFTEN ☐	CONSTANT ☐
LOSS OF BLADDER/BOWEL CONTROL	NOT AT ALL ☐ SEVERAL TIMES ☐	OFTEN ☐	CONSTANT ☐
SUDDEN SEVERE PAIN	NOT AT ALL ☐ SEVERAL TIMES ☐	OFTEN ☐	CONSTANT ☐
NEW SWELLING/REDNESS	NOT AT ALL ☐ SEVERAL TIMES ☐	OFTEN ☐	CONSTANT ☐

IT IS ESSENTIAL TO BRING THESE RESULTS UP WITH YOUR HEALTHCARE PROVIDER AS SOON AS POSSIBLE.

FLARE PATTERN CHECK-IN

During this week, I had flares that felt:

SUDDEN	NOT AT ALL ☐ SEVERAL TIMES ☐	OFTEN ☐
SLOW-BUILDING	NOT AT ALL ☐ SEVERAL TIMES ☐	OFTEN ☐
TRIGGERED	NOT AT ALL ☐ SEVERAL TIMES ☐	OFTEN ☐
RANDOM	NOT AT ALL ☐ SEVERAL TIMES ☐	OFTEN ☐
WORSE THAN USUAL	NOT AT ALL ☐ SEVERAL TIMES ☐	OFTEN ☐
UNUSUAL COMPARED TO TYPICAL FLARES	NOT AT ALL ☐ SEVERAL TIMES ☐	OFTEN ☐

DURATION OF FLARES _____

Notes

_____

_____

_____

_____

WEEKLY SUMMARY
PATTERNS & NOTES

Week Of:

Patterns / Similarities On Good Days

○ _____
○ _____
○ _____
○ _____
○ _____

Patterns / Similarities On Bad Days

○ _____
○ _____
○ _____
○ _____
○ _____

Things That Improved Symptoms

○ _____
○ _____
○ _____
○ _____
○ _____

WEEKLY SUMMARY
PATTERNS & NOTES

Week Of:

Most Common Symptoms

○ _____
○ _____
○ _____
○ _____
○ _____

Most Common Triggers

○ _____
○ _____
○ _____
○ _____
○ _____

Symptom Timing Patterns
When do your symptoms tend to be at their worst?

MORNING ☐   AFTER MEALS ☐
AFTERNOON ☐   AFTER PHYSICAL ACTIVITY ☐
EVENING ☐   HORMONE FLUCTUATIONS ☐
NIGHT ☐   DURING STRESS ☐
UPON WAKING ☐   DURING WEATHER CHANGES ☐

NOTES
_____
_____
_____
_____
_____
_____
_____
_____
_____
_____
_____
_____
_____
_____
_____
_____

Overall Effectiveness Of Treatment This Week

○———○———○———○———○
LOW   HIGH

Overall Stress This Week

○———○———○———○———○
LOW   HIGH

Overall Sleep This Week

○———○———○———○———○
LOW   HIGH

IMPORTANT NOTES

NEW WEEK CHECK-IN
PATTERNS & NOTES

How Did Last Week Go Overall?   ○———○———○———○———○

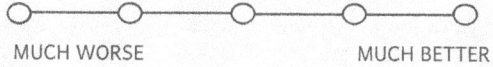

MUCH WORSE   MUCH BETTER

Any Clear Patterns Or Triggers?   New Things You're Trying This Week

○ _____   ○ _____
○ _____   ○ _____
○ _____   ○ _____
○ _____   ○ _____
○ _____   ○ _____

Changes To Medication/Supplements?   YES ☐   NO ☐

NOTE: _____

Changes To Treatment/Therapies?   YES ☐   NO ☐

NOTE: _____

Emotional & Mental Health Check-In

HOW ARE YOU FEELING HEADING INTO THIS WEEK? ANYTHING WEIGHING ON YOU?

_____

_____

_____

_____

_____

_____

DAILY SYMPTOM TRACKER

Date:

Sleep QUALITY (1-10) _____ LENGTH _____

Flare Status SUDDEN ☐ TRIGGERED ☐ SLOW BUILDING ☐ RANDOM ☐

NO FLARE ○ ○ ○ ○ ○ SEVERE FLAIR

MILD   MODERATE

Weather HOT ☐ DRY ☐ HUMID ☐
RAIN ☐ STORM ☐ COLD ☐

SUSPECTED TRIGGER _____

Today's Symptoms

	LOW	HIGH
FEVER	○—○—○—○—○	
FATIGUE	○—○—○—○—○	

Systemic

DIZZINESS	☐	NIGHT SWEATS	☐
WEIGHT CHANGE	☐	FLUE-LIKE	☐
CHILLS	☐	BRAIN FOG	☐

Pain & Inflammation

JOINT PAIN	☐	JOINT SWELLING	☐
STIFFNESS	☐	MUSCLE ACHES	☐
WEAKNESS	☐	BACK PAIN	☐
NERVE PAIN	☐	MIGRAINES	☐

Thyroid-like

TREMORS	☐	HEART PALPITATIONS	☐
HEAT/COLD SENSITITVITY	☐	WEIGHT SHIFT	☐
CHILLS	☐	NECK PAIN	☐

Skin, Hair & Nails

RASH	☐	REDNESS/FLUSHING	☐
HIVES	☐	SENSITITY TO SUN	☐
ITCHING	☐	BRITTLE NAILS	☐
HAIR LOSS	☐	DRY SKIN	☐

Respiratory

CHEST PAIN	☐	CHRONIC COUGH	☐
SHORTNESS OF BREATH	☐		

Kidneys

FOAMY URINE	☐	SWELLING IN LEGS / ANKLES	☐
DARK URINE	☐	BLOODY URINE	☐

Digestive / GI

NAUSEA	☐	STOMACH PAINS	☐
VOMITING	☐	FOOD REACTIONS	☐
DIARRHEA	☐	APPETITE LOSS	☐
CONSTIPATION	☐	BLOATING	☐

Vascular

NUMB FINGERS/TOES	☐	RAYNAUD'S COLOR CHANGES	☐

DAILY SYMPTOM TRACKER

Date:

Stress Level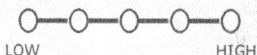
LOW   HIGH

Pain's Impact On Today's Function
Today pain affected my ability to:

DRIVE ☐   WORK ☐   SOCIALIZE ☐

COOK ☐   LIFT/CARRY ☐   LEAVE THE HOUSE ☐

WALK ☐   CARE FOR SELF ☐   SIT/LAY DOWN ☐

Symptom Changes Throughout The Day

CONSISTENT ☐   WORSE AT NIGHT ☐

COMES IN WAVES ☐   PAIN FLARE ☐

WORSE IN MORNING ☐

Notes

_____

_____

_____

_____

_____

_____

_____

_____

Today's Water Intake

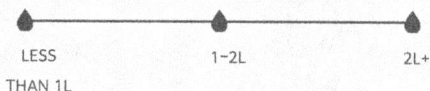
LESS THAN 1L   1–2L   2L+

Food & Immune Response

DID YOU EAT ANYTHING NEW TODAY?
YES ☐   NO ☐

Impact On Symptoms

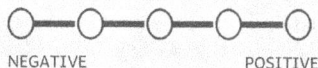
NEGATIVE   POSITIVE

Notes

_____

_____

_____

_____

_____

_____

Activity Overview

REST DAY ☐   LIGHT MOVEMENT ☐

MODERATE ACTIVITY ☐   HEAVY ACTIVITY ☐

WORSE   BETTER
Effect On Pain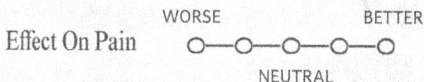
NEUTRAL

DAILY SYMPTOM TRACKER

Date:

Sleep QUALITY (1-10) _____ LENGTH _____

Flare Status
SUDDEN ☐   TRIGGERED ☐
SLOW BUILDING ☐   RANDOM ☐

NO FLARE ○ ○ ○ ○ ○ SEVERE FLAIR
MILD   MODERATE

SUSPECTED TRIGGER _____

Weather
HOT ☐   DRY ☐   HUMID ☐
RAIN ☐   STORM ☐   COLD ☐

Today's Symptoms

Systemic

	LOW	HIGH
FEVER	○—○—○—○—○	
FATIGUE	○—○—○—○—○	

DIZZINESS ☐   NIGHT SWEATS ☐
WEIGHT CHANGE ☐   FLUE-LIKE ☐
CHILLS ☐   BRAIN FOG ☐

Pain & Inflammation

JOINT PAIN ☐   JOINT SWELLING ☐
STIFFNESS ☐   MUSCLE ACHES ☐
WEAKNESS ☐   BACK PAIN ☐
NERVE PAIN ☐   MIGRAINES ☐

Thyroid-like

TREMORS ☐   HEART PALPITATIONS ☐
HEAT/COLD SENSITITVITY ☐   WEIGHT SHIFT ☐
CHILLS ☐   NECK PAIN ☐

Skin, Hair & Nails

RASH ☐   REDNESS/FLUSHING ☐
HIVES ☐   SENSITITY TO SUN ☐
ITCHING ☐   BRITTLE NAILS ☐
HAIR LOSS ☐   DRY SKIN ☐

Respiratory

CHEST PAIN ☐   CHRONIC COUGH ☐
SHORTNESS OF BREATH ☐

Kidneys

FOAMY URINE ☐   SWELLING IN LEGS / ANKLES ☐
DARK URINE ☐   BLOODY URINE ☐

Digestive / GI

NAUSEA ☐   STOMACH PAINS ☐
VOMITING ☐   FOOD REACTIONS ☐
DIARRHEA ☐   APPETITE LOSS ☐
CONSTIPATION ☐   BLOATING ☐

Vascular

NUMB FINGERS/TOES ☐   RAYNAUD'S COLOR CHANGES ☐

DAILY SYMPTOM TRACKER

Date:

Stress Level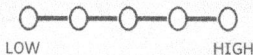
          LOW   HIGH

Pain's Impact On Today's Function
Today pain affected my ability to:

DRIVE ☐   WORK ☐   SOCIALIZE ☐

COOK ☐   LIFT/CARRY ☐   LEAVE THE HOUSE ☐

WALK ☐   CARE FOR SELF ☐   SIT/LAY DOWN ☐

Symptom Changes Throughout The Day

CONSISTENT ☐   WORSE AT NIGHT ☐

COMES IN WAVES ☐   PAIN FLARE ☐

WORSE IN MORNING ☐

Notes

_____

_____

_____

_____

_____

_____

_____

_____

Today's Water Intake
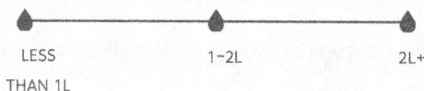
LESS THAN 1L   1–2L   2L+

Food & Immune Response

DID YOU EAT ANYTHING NEW TODAY?

YES ☐   NO ☐

Impact On Symptoms
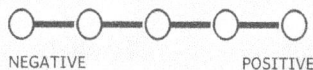
NEGATIVE   POSITIVE

Notes

_____

_____

_____

_____

_____

_____

Activity Overview

REST DAY ☐   LIGHT MOVEMENT ☐

MODERATE ACTIVITY ☐   HEAVY ACTIVITY ☐

WORSE   BETTER

Effect On Pain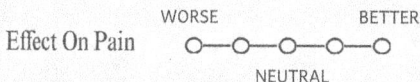
NEUTRAL

DAILY SYMPTOM TRACKER

Date:

Sleep QUALITY (1-10)_____ LENGTH _____

Flare Status
SUDDEN ☐ TRIGGERED ☐
SLOW BUILDING ☐ RANDOM ☐

NO FLARE ◯ ◯ ◯ ◯ ◯ SEVERE FLAIR
MILD MODERATE

Weather
HOT ☐ DRY ☐ HUMID ☐
RAIN ☐ STORM ☐ COLD ☐

SUSPECTED TRIGGER _____

Today's Symptoms

	LOW	HIGH
FEVER	◯—◯—◯—◯—◯	
FATIGUE	◯—◯—◯—◯—◯	

Pain & Inflammation

JOINT PAIN ☐	JOINT SWELLING ☐
STIFFNESS ☐	MUSCLE ACHES ☐
WEAKNESS ☐	BACK PAIN ☐
NERVE PAIN ☐	MIGRAINES ☐

Skin, Hair & Nails

RASH ☐	REDNESS/FLUSHING ☐
HIVES ☐	SENSITITITY TO SUN ☐
ITCHING ☐	BRITTLE NAILS ☐
HAIR LOSS ☐	DRY SKIN ☐

Digestive / GI

NAUSEA ☐	STOMACH PAINS ☐
VOMITING ☐	FOOD REACTIONS ☐
DIARRHEA ☐	APPETITE LOSS ☐
CONSTIPATION ☐	BLOATING ☐

Systemic

DIZZINESS ☐	NIGHT SWEATS ☐
WEIGHT CHANGE ☐	FLUE-LIKE ☐
CHILLS ☐	BRAIN FOG ☐

Thyroid-like

TREMORS ☐	HEART PALPITATIONS ☐
HEAT/COLD SENSITITVITY ☐	WEIGHT SHIFT ☐
CHILLS ☐	NECK PAIN ☐

Respiratory

CHEST PAIN ☐	CHRONIC COUGH ☐
SHORTNESS OF BREATH ☐	

Kidneys

FOAMY URINE ☐	SWELLING IN LEGS / ANKLES ☐
DARK URINE ☐	BLOODY URINE ☐

Vascular

NUMB FINGERS/TOES ☐	RAYNAUD'S COLOR CHANGES ☐

DAILY SYMPTOM TRACKER

Date:

Stress Level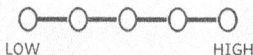
LOW   HIGH

Today's Water Intake

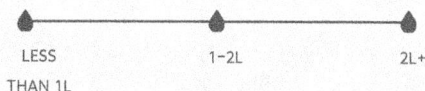

LESS   1–2L   2L+
THAN 1L

Pain's Impact On Today's Function

Today pain affected my ability to:

DRIVE	☐	WORK	☐	SOCIALIZE	☐
COOK	☐	LIFT/CARRY	☐	LEAVE THE HOUSE	☐
WALK	☐	CARE FOR SELF	☐	SIT/LAY DOWN	☐

Food & Immune Response

DID YOU EAT ANYTHING NEW TODAY?

YES ☐   NO ☐

Impact On Symptoms

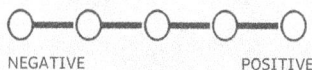

NEGATIVE   POSITIVE

Notes

_____

_____

_____

_____

_____

_____

Symptom Changes Throughout The Day

CONSISTENT	☐	WORSE AT NIGHT	☐
COMES IN WAVES	☐	PAIN FLARE	☐
WORSE IN MORNING	☐		

Notes

_____

_____

_____

_____

_____

_____

_____

Activity Overview

REST DAY	☐	LIGHT MOVEMENT	☐
MODERATE ACTIVITY	☐	HEAVY ACTIVITY	☐

WORSE   BETTER

Effect On Pain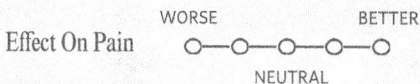

NEUTRAL

DAILY SYMPTOM TRACKER

Date:

Sleep QUALITY (1-10) _____ LENGTH _____

Flare Status
SUDDEN ☐ TRIGGERED ☐
SLOW BUILDING ☐ RANDOM ☐

NO FLARE ○ ○ ○ ○ ○ SEVERE FLAIR
MILD   MODERATE

Weather
HOT ☐ DRY ☐ HUMID ☐
RAIN ☐ STORM ☐ COLD ☐

SUSPECTED TRIGGER _____

Today's Symptoms

LOW   HIGH

FEVER   ○—○—○—○—○

FATIGUE   ○—○—○—○—○

Pain & Inflammation

JOINT PAIN ☐   JOINT SWELLING ☐

STIFFNESS ☐   MUSCLE ACHES ☐

WEAKNESS ☐   BACK PAIN ☐

NERVE PAIN ☐   MIGRAINES ☐

Skin, Hair & Nails

RASH ☐   REDNESS/FLUSHING ☐

HIVES ☐   SENSITITY TO SUN ☐

ITCHING ☐   BRITTLE NAILS ☐

HAIR LOSS ☐   DRY SKIN ☐

Digestive / GI

NAUSEA ☐   STOMACH PAINS ☐

VOMITING ☐   FOOD REACTIONS ☐

DIARRHEA ☐   APPETITE LOSS ☐

CONSTIPATION ☐   BLOATING ☐

Systemic

DIZZINESS ☐   NIGHT SWEATS ☐

WEIGHT CHANGE ☐   FLUE-LIKE ☐

CHILLS ☐   BRAIN FOG ☐

Thyroid-like

TREMORS ☐   HEART PALPITATIONS ☐

HEAT/COLD SENSITITVITY ☐   WEIGHT SHIFT ☐

CHILLS ☐   NECK PAIN ☐

Respiratory

CHEST PAIN ☐   CHRONIC COUGH ☐

SHORTNESS OF BREATH ☐

Kidneys

FOAMY URINE ☐   SWELLING IN LEGS / ANKLES ☐

DARK URINE ☐   BLOODY URINE ☐

Vascular

NUMB FINGERS/TOES ☐   RAYNAUD'S COLOR CHANGES ☐

DAILY SYMPTOM TRACKER

Date:

Stress Level

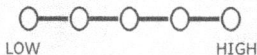

LOW   HIGH

Pain's Impact On Today's Function

Today pain affected my ability to:

DRIVE ☐   WORK ☐   SOCIALIZE ☐

COOK ☐   LIFT/CARRY ☐   LEAVE THE HOUSE ☐

WALK ☐   CARE FOR SELF ☐   SIT/LAY DOWN ☐

Symptom Changes Throughout The Day

CONSISTENT ☐   WORSE AT NIGHT ☐

COMES IN WAVES ☐   PAIN FLARE ☐

WORSE IN MORNING ☐

Notes

_____

_____

_____

_____

_____

_____

_____

Today's Water Intake

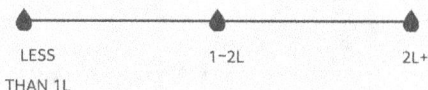

LESS THAN 1L   1–2L   2L+

Food & Immune Response

DID YOU EAT ANYTHING NEW TODAY?

YES ☐   NO ☐

Impact On Symptoms

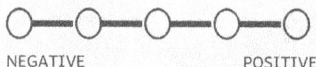

NEGATIVE   POSITIVE

Notes

_____

_____

_____

_____

_____

_____

Activity Overview

REST DAY ☐   LIGHT MOVEMENT ☐

MODERATE ACTIVITY ☐   HEAVY ACTIVITY ☐

Effect On Pain

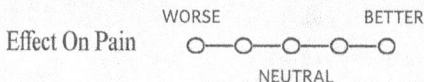

WORSE   BETTER

NEUTRAL

DAILY SYMPTOM TRACKER

Date:

Sleep QUALITY (1-10) _____ LENGTH _____

Flare Status
SUDDEN ☐ TRIGGERED ☐
SLOW BUILDING ☐ RANDOM ☐

NO FLARE ○ ○ ○ ○ ○ SEVERE FLAIR
MILD   MODERATE

Weather
HOT ☐ DRY ☐ HUMID ☐
RAIN ☐ STORM ☐ COLD ☐

SUSPECTED TRIGGER _____

Today's Symptoms

LOW   HIGH

FEVER ○—○—○—○—○

FATIGUE ○—○—○—○—○

Systemic

DIZZINESS ☐   NIGHT SWEATS ☐

WEIGHT CHANGE ☐   FLUE-LIKE ☐

CHILLS ☐   BRAIN FOG ☐

Pain & Inflammation

JOINT PAIN ☐   JOINT SWELLING ☐

STIFFNESS ☐   MUSCLE ACHES ☐

WEAKNESS ☐   BACK PAIN ☐

NERVE PAIN ☐   MIGRAINES ☐

Thyroid-like

TREMORS ☐   HEART PALPITATIONS ☐

HEAT/COLD SENSITITVITY ☐   WEIGHT SHIFT ☐

CHILLS ☐   NECK PAIN ☐

Skin, Hair & Nails

RASH ☐   REDNESS/FLUSHING ☐

HIVES ☐   SENSITITIY TO SUN ☐

ITCHING ☐   BRITTLE NAILS ☐

HAIR LOSS ☐   DRY SKIN ☐

Respiratory

CHEST PAIN ☐   CHRONIC COUGH ☐

SHORTNESS OF BREATH ☐

Kidneys

FOAMY URINE ☐   SWELLING IN LEGS / ANKLES ☐

DARK URINE ☐   BLOODY URINE ☐

Digestive / GI

NAUSEA ☐   STOMACH PAINS ☐

VOMITING ☐   FOOD REACTIONS ☐

DIARRHEA ☐   APPETITE LOSS ☐

CONSTIPATION ☐   BLOATING ☐

Vascular

NUMB FINGERS/TOES ☐   RAYNAUD'S COLOR CHANGES ☐

DAILY SYMPTOM TRACKER

Date:

Stress Level

O—O—O—O—O
LOW   HIGH

Pain's Impact On Today's Function

Today pain affected my ability to:

DRIVE ☐   WORK ☐   SOCIALIZE ☐

COOK ☐   LIFT/CARRY ☐   LEAVE THE ☐
                             HOUSE

WALK ☐   CARE FOR ☐   SIT/LAY ☐
            SELF   DOWN

Symptom Changes Throughout The Day

CONSISTENT ☐   WORSE AT NIGHT ☐

COMES IN WAVES ☐   PAIN FLARE ☐

WORSE IN MORNING ☐

Notes

_____

_____

_____

_____

_____

_____

_____

_____

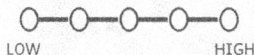

Today's Water Intake

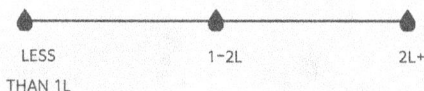

◆————————◆————————◆
LESS   1–2L   2L+
THAN 1L

Food & Immune Response

DID YOU EAT ANYTHING NEW TODAY?

YES ☐   NO ☐

Impact On Symptoms

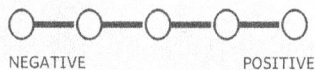

O—O—O—O—O
NEGATIVE   POSITIVE

Notes

_____

_____

_____

_____

_____

_____

Activity Overview

REST DAY ☐   LIGHT MOVEMENT ☐

MODERATE ACTIVITY ☐   HEAVY ACTIVITY ☐

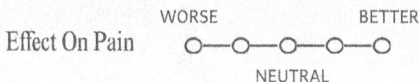

                WORSE   BETTER
Effect On Pain O—O—O—O—O
                        NEUTRAL

DAILY SYMPTOM TRACKER

Date:

Sleep QUALITY (1-10) _____ LENGTH _____

Flare Status
SUDDEN ☐ TRIGGERED ☐
SLOW BUILDING ☐ RANDOM ☐

NO FLARE ○ ○ ○ ○ ○ SEVERE FLAIR
MILD   MODERATE

Weather
HOT ☐ DRY ☐ HUMID ☐
RAIN ☐ STORM ☐ COLD ☐

SUSPECTED TRIGGER _____

Today's Symptoms

LOW —————— HIGH

FEVER   ○—○—○—○—○
FATIGUE ○—○—○—○—○

Systemic

DIZZINESS ☐   NIGHT SWEATS ☐
WEIGHT CHANGE ☐   FLUE-LIKE ☐
CHILLS ☐   BRAIN FOG ☐

Pain & Inflammation

JOINT PAIN ☐   JOINT SWELLING ☐
STIFFNESS ☐   MUSCLE ACHES ☐
WEAKNESS ☐   BACK PAIN ☐
NERVE PAIN ☐   MIGRAINES ☐

Thyroid-like

TREMORS ☐   HEART PALPITATIONS ☐
HEAT/COLD SENSITITVITY ☐   WEIGHT SHIFT ☐
CHILLS ☐   NECK PAIN ☐

Skin, Hair & Nails

RASH ☐   REDNESS/FLUSHING ☐
HIVES ☐   SENSITITITY TO SUN ☐
ITCHING ☐   BRITTLE NAILS ☐
HAIR LOSS ☐   DRY SKIN ☐

Respiratory

CHEST PAIN ☐   CHRONIC COUGH ☐
SHORTNESS OF BREATH ☐

Kidneys

FOAMY URINE ☐   SWELLING IN LEGS / ANKLES ☐
DARK URINE ☐   BLOODY URINE ☐

Digestive / GI

NAUSEA ☐   STOMACH PAINS ☐
VOMITING ☐   FOOD REACTIONS ☐
DIARRHEA ☐   APPETITE LOSS ☐
CONSTIPATION ☐   BLOATING ☐

Vascular

NUMB FINGERS/TOES ☐   RAYNAUD'S COLOR CHANGES ☐

DAILY SYMPTOM TRACKER

Date:

Stress Level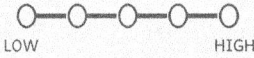
LOW   HIGH

Pain's Impact On Today's Function
Today pain affected my ability to:

DRIVE ☐   WORK ☐   SOCIALIZE ☐

COOK ☐   LIFT/CARRY ☐   LEAVE THE HOUSE ☐

WALK ☐   CARE FOR SELF ☐   SIT/LAY DOWN ☐

Symptom Changes Throughout The Day

CONSISTENT ☐   WORSE AT NIGHT ☐

COMES IN WAVES ☐   PAIN FLARE ☐

WORSE IN MORNING ☐

Notes

_____

_____

_____

_____

_____

_____

_____

_____

Today's Water Intake

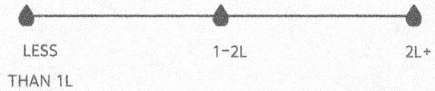
LESS THAN 1L   1–2L   2L+

Food & Immune Response

DID YOU EAT ANYTHING NEW TODAY?

YES ☐   NO ☐

Impact On Symptoms

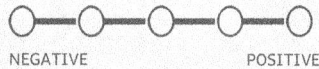
NEGATIVE   POSITIVE

Notes

_____

_____

_____

_____

_____

_____

Activity Overview

REST DAY ☐   LIGHT MOVEMENT ☐

MODERATE ACTIVITY ☐   HEAVY ACTIVITY ☐

WORSE   BETTER

Effect On Pain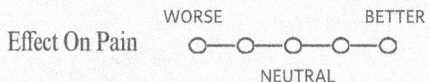
NEUTRAL

DAILY SYMPTOM TRACKER

Date:

Sleep
QUALITY (1–10) _____ LENGTH _____

Flare Status
SUDDEN ☐   TRIGGERED ☐
SLOW BUILDING ☐   RANDOM ☐

NO FLARE ○   ○   ○   ○   ○ SEVERE FLAIR
MILD   MODERATE

SUSPECTED TRIGGER _____

Weather
HOT ☐   DRY ☐   HUMID ☐
RAIN ☐   STORM ☐   COLD ☐

Today's Symptoms

Systemic

DIZZINESS ☐   NIGHT SWEATS ☐
WEIGHT CHANGE ☐   FLUE–LIKE ☐
CHILLS ☐   BRAIN FOG ☐

LOW ○—○—○—○—○ HIGH
FEVER
FATIGUE ○—○—○—○—○

Pain & Inflammation

JOINT PAIN ☐   JOINT SWELLING ☐
STIFFNESS ☐   MUSCLE ACHES ☐
WEAKNESS ☐   BACK PAIN ☐
NERVE PAIN ☐   MIGRAINES ☐

Thyroid-like

TREMORS ☐   HEART PALPITATIONS ☐
HEAT/COLD SENSITITVITY ☐   WEIGHT SHIFT ☐
CHILLS ☐   NECK PAIN ☐

Skin, Hair & Nails

RASH ☐   REDNESS/FLUSHING ☐
HIVES ☐   SENSITITY TO SUN ☐
ITCHING ☐   BRITTLE NAILS ☐
HAIR LOSS ☐   DRY SKIN ☐

Respiratory

CHEST PAIN ☐   CHRONIC COUGH ☐
SHORTNESS OF BREATH ☐

Kidneys

FOAMY URINE ☐   SWELLING IN LEGS / ANKLES ☐
DARK URINE ☐   BLOODY URINE ☐

Digestive / GI

NAUSEA ☐   STOMACH PAINS ☐
VOMITING ☐   FOOD REACTIONS ☐
DIARRHEA ☐   APPETITE LOSS ☐
CONSTIPATION ☐   BLOATING ☐

Vascular

NUMB FINGERS/TOES ☐   RAYNAUD'S COLOR CHANGES ☐

DAILY SYMPTOM TRACKER

Date:

Stress Level O—O—O—O—O
              LOW   HIGH

Pain's Impact On Today's Function
Today pain affected my ability to:

DRIVE ☐   WORK ☐   SOCIALIZE ☐

COOK ☐   LIFT/CARRY ☐   LEAVE THE HOUSE ☐

WALK ☐   CARE FOR SELF ☐   SIT/LAY DOWN ☐

Symptom Changes Throughout The Day

CONSISTENT ☐   WORSE AT NIGHT ☐

COMES IN WAVES ☐   PAIN FLARE ☐

WORSE IN MORNING ☐

Notes

_____

_____

_____

_____

_____

_____

_____

_____

Today's Water Intake

◆————————◆————————◆
LESS THAN 1L   1–2L   2L+

Food & Immune Response

DID YOU EAT ANYTHING NEW TODAY?

YES ☐   NO ☐

Impact On Symptoms

O—O—O—O—O
NEGATIVE   POSITIVE

Notes

_____

_____

_____

_____

_____

_____

Activity Overview

REST DAY ☐   LIGHT MOVEMENT ☐

MODERATE ACTIVITY ☐   HEAVY ACTIVITY ☐

Effect On Pain   WORSE   BETTER
                   O—O—O—O—O
                         NEUTRAL

IMPORTANT NOTES

WEEKLY SUMMARY

Week Of:

Sleep	Overall Feelings
QUALITY (1-10) _____	MOOD (1-10) _____ MENTAL CLARITY (1-10) _____ ENERGY (1-10) _____ IMPACT FROM WEATHER (1-10) _____

Autoimmune Flare Snapshot

This week:

I EXPERIENCED UNUSUAL FATIGUE	NOT AT ALL ☐	SEVERAL TIMES ☐	OFTEN ☐	CONSTANT ☐
MY PAIN WAS	LOW ☐	MILD ☐	WORSE ☐	CONSTANT ☐
I HAD MORNING STIFFNESS	NOT AT ALL ☐	30 MINUTES ☐	30-60 ☐	OVER 60 ☐
MY SYMPTOMS WORSENED WITH ACTIVITY	NOT AT ALL ☐	SEVERAL TIMES ☐	OFTEN ☐	CONSTANT ☐
MY SYMPTOMS WORSENED WITH REST	NOT AT ALL ☐	SEVERAL TIMES ☐	OFTEN ☐	CONSTANT ☐
I HAD FLU-LIKE SENSATIONS	NOT AT ALL ☐	SEVERAL TIMES ☐	OFTEN ☐	CONSTANT ☐

FATIGUE & ENERGY CHECK-IN

This week made feel:

FEELING "POISONED" OR SICK	NOT AT ALL ☐	SEVERAL TIMES ☐	OFTEN ☐	CONSTANT ☐
EXHAUSTION AFTER SMALL TASKS	NOT AT ALL ☐	SEVERAL TIMES ☐	OFTEN ☐	CONSTANT ☐
FEELING TIRED EVEN AFTER RESTING	NOT AT ALL ☐	SEVERAL TIMES ☐	OFTEN ☐	CONSTANT ☐
MUSCLES FEELING WEAK OR "HEAVY"	NOT AT ALL ☐	SEVERAL TIMES ☐	OFTEN ☐	CONSTANT ☐
NEEDING NAPS TO FUNCTION	NOT AT ALL ☐	SEVERAL TIMES ☐	OFTEN ☐	CONSTANT ☐
BRAIN FOG INTERFERING WITH THINKING	NOT AT ALL ☐	SEVERAL TIMES ☐	OFTEN ☐	CONSTANT ☐

MOBILITY CHECK-IN

During this week, how often did you experience:

STIFFNESS IN THE MORNING	NOT AT ALL ☐	SEVERAL TIMES ☐	OFTEN ☐	CONSTANT ☐
DIFFICULTY GETTING OUT OF BED	NOT AT ALL ☐	SEVERAL TIMES ☐	OFTEN ☐	CONSTANT ☐
REDUCED RANGE OF MOTION	NOT AT ALL ☐	SEVERAL TIMES ☐	OFTEN ☐	CONSTANT ☐
TROUBLE GRIPPING OR LIFTING	NOT AT ALL ☐	SEVERAL TIMES ☐	OFTEN ☐	CONSTANT ☐
SLOWER WALKING SPEED	NOT AT ALL ☐	SEVERAL TIMES ☐	OFTEN ☐	CONSTANT ☐
FEELING UNSTABLE OR WEAK	NOT AT ALL ☐	SEVERAL TIMES ☐	OFTEN ☐	CONSTANT ☐
NEEDED MOBILITY AIDS	NOT AT ALL ☐	SEVERAL TIMES ☐	OFTEN ☐	CONSTANT ☐

WEEKLY SUMMARY

Week Of:

Sleep	Overall Feelings		
QUALITY (1-10) _____	MOOD (1-10) _____	MENTAL CLARITY (1-10) _____	
	ENERGY (1-10) _____	IMPACT FROM WEATHER (1-10) _____	

RED FLAG CHECK-IN

During this week, did you notice:

NEW NUMBNESS	NOT AT ALL ☐ SEVERAL TIMES ☐	OFTEN ☐	CONSTANT ☐
NEW WEAKNESS	NOT AT ALL ☐ SEVERAL TIMES ☐	OFTEN ☐	CONSTANT ☐
PAIN THAT WOKE ME FROM SLEEP	NOT AT ALL ☐ SEVERAL TIMES ☐	OFTEN ☐	CONSTANT ☐
LOSS OF BLADDER/BOWEL CONTROL	NOT AT ALL ☐ SEVERAL TIMES ☐	OFTEN ☐	CONSTANT ☐
SUDDEN SEVERE PAIN	NOT AT ALL ☐ SEVERAL TIMES ☐	OFTEN ☐	CONSTANT ☐
NEW SWELLING/REDNESS	NOT AT ALL ☐ SEVERAL TIMES ☐	OFTEN ☐	CONSTANT ☐

IT IS ESSENTIAL TO BRING THESE RESULTS UP WITH YOUR HEALTHCARE PROVIDER AS SOON AS POSSIBLE.

FLARE PATTERN CHECK-IN

During this week, I had flares that felt:

SUDDEN	NOT AT ALL ☐	SEVERAL TIMES ☐	OFTEN ☐
SLOW-BUILDING	NOT AT ALL ☐	SEVERAL TIMES ☐	OFTEN ☐
TRIGGERED	NOT AT ALL ☐	SEVERAL TIMES ☐	OFTEN ☐
RANDOM	NOT AT ALL ☐	SEVERAL TIMES ☐	OFTEN ☐
WORSE THAN USUAL	NOT AT ALL ☐	SEVERAL TIMES ☐	OFTEN ☐
UNUSUAL COMPARED TO TYPICAL FLARES	NOT AT ALL ☐	SEVERAL TIMES ☐	OFTEN ☐

DURATION OF FLARES _____

Notes

_____

_____

_____

_____

WEEKLY SUMMARY
PATTERNS & NOTES

Week Of:

Patterns / Similarities On Good Days

○ _____
○ _____
○ _____
○ _____
○ _____

Patterns / Similarities On Bad Days

○ _____
○ _____
○ _____
○ _____
○ _____

Things That Improved Symptoms

○ _____
○ _____
○ _____
○ _____
○ _____

WEEKLY SUMMARY
PATTERNS & NOTES

Week Of:

Most Common Symptoms

- _____
- _____
- _____
- _____
- _____

Most Common Triggers

- _____
- _____
- _____
- _____
- _____

Symptom Timing Patterns
When do your symptoms tend to be at their worst?

MORNING ☐   AFTER MEALS ☐

AFTERNOON ☐   AFTER PHYSICAL ACTIVITY ☐

EVENING ☐   HORMONE FLUCTUATIONS ☐

NIGHT ☐   DURING STRESS ☐

UPON WAKING ☐   DURING WEATHER CHANGES ☐

NOTES

_____

_____

_____

_____

_____

_____

_____

_____

_____

_____

_____

_____

_____

_____

_____

_____

Overall Effectiveness Of Treatment This Week

○———○———○———○———○

LOW   HIGH

Overall Stress This Week

○———○———○———○———○

LOW   HIGH

Overall Sleep This Week

○———○———○———○———○

LOW   HIGH

IMPORTANT NOTES

NEW WEEK CHECK-IN
PATTERNS & NOTES

How Did Last Week Go Overall? ○——○——○——○——○

MUCH WORSE   MUCH BETTER

Any Clear Patterns Or Triggers?

○ _____
○ _____
○ _____
○ _____
○ _____

New Things You're Trying This Week

○ _____
○ _____
○ _____
○ _____
○ _____

Changes To Medication/Supplements?   YES ☐   NO ☐

NOTE: _____

Changes To Treatment/Therapies?   YES ☐   NO ☐

NOTE: _____

Emotional & Mental Health Check-In

HOW ARE YOU FEELING HEADING INTO THIS WEEK? ANYTHING WEIGHING ON YOU?

_____
_____
_____
_____
_____
_____

DAILY SYMPTOM TRACKER

Date:

Sleep QUALITY (1-10) _____ LENGTH _____

Flare Status
SUDDEN ☐ TRIGGERED ☐
SLOW BUILDING ☐ RANDOM ☐

NO FLARE ○ ○ ○ ○ ○ SEVERE FLAIR
MILD MODERATE

SUSPECTED TRIGGER _____

Weather
HOT ☐ DRY ☐ HUMID ☐
RAIN ☐ STORM ☐ COLD ☐

Today's Symptoms

	LOW	HIGH
FEVER	○—○—○—○—○	
FATIGUE	○—○—○—○—○	

Systemic

DIZZINESS	☐	NIGHT SWEATS	☐
WEIGHT CHANGE	☐	FLUE-LIKE	☐
CHILLS	☐	BRAIN FOG	☐

Pain & Inflammation

JOINT PAIN	☐	JOINT SWELLING	☐
STIFFNESS	☐	MUSCLE ACHES	☐
WEAKNESS	☐	BACK PAIN	☐
NERVE PAIN	☐	MIGRAINES	☐

Thyroid-like

TREMORS	☐	HEART PALPITATIONS	☐
HEAT/COLD SENSITITVITY	☐	WEIGHT SHIFT	☐
CHILLS	☐	NECK PAIN	☐

Skin, Hair & Nails

RASH	☐	REDNESS/FLUSHING	☐
HIVES	☐	SENSITITY TO SUN	☐
ITCHING	☐	BRITTLE NAILS	☐
HAIR LOSS	☐	DRY SKIN	☐

Respiratory

CHEST PAIN	☐	CHRONIC COUGH	☐
SHORTNESS OF BREATH	☐		

Kidneys

FOAMY URINE	☐	SWELLING IN LEGS / ANKLES	☐
DARK URINE	☐	BLOODY URINE	☐

Digestive / GI

NAUSEA	☐	STOMACH PAINS	☐
VOMITING	☐	FOOD REACTIONS	☐
DIARRHEA	☐	APPETITE LOSS	☐
CONSTIPATION	☐	BLOATING	☐

Vascular

NUMB FINGERS/TOES	☐	RAYNAUD'S COLOR CHANGES	☐

DAILY SYMPTOM TRACKER

Date:

Stress Level O—O—O—O—O
LOW   HIGH

Today's Water Intake

🌢————————🌢————————🌢
LESS   1–2L   2L+
THAN 1L

Pain's Impact On Today's Function
Today pain affected my ability to:

DRIVE ☐   WORK ☐   SOCIALIZE ☐

COOK ☐   LIFT/CARRY ☐   LEAVE THE ☐
                                        HOUSE

WALK ☐   CARE FOR ☐   SIT/LAY ☐
                SELF   DOWN

Food & Immune Response

DID YOU EAT ANYTHING NEW TODAY?

YES ☐   NO ☐

Impact On Symptoms

O—O—O—O—O
NEGATIVE   POSITIVE

Notes

_____

_____

_____

_____

_____

_____

_____

Symptom Changes Throughout The Day

CONSISTENT ☐   WORSE AT NIGHT ☐

COMES IN WAVES ☐   PAIN FLARE ☐

WORSE IN MORNING ☐

Notes

_____

_____

_____

_____

_____

_____

_____

_____

_____

_____

Activity Overview

REST DAY ☐   LIGHT MOVEMENT ☐

MODERATE ACTIVITY ☐   HEAVY ACTIVITY ☐

                        WORSE   BETTER
Effect On Pain O—O—O—O—O
                              NEUTRAL

DAILY SYMPTOM TRACKER

Date:

Sleep QUALITY (1-10) _____ LENGTH _____

Flare Status
SUDDEN ☐ TRIGGERED ☐
SLOW BUILDING ☐ RANDOM ☐

NO FLARE ○ ○ ○ ○ ○ SEVERE FLAIR
MILD   MODERATE

SUSPECTED TRIGGER _____

Weather
HOT ☐ DRY ☐ HUMID ☐
RAIN ☐ STORM ☐ COLD ☐

Today's Symptoms

	LOW	HIGH
FEVER	○—○—○—○—○	
FATIGUE	○—○—○—○—○	

Systemic

DIZZINESS	☐	NIGHT SWEATS	☐
WEIGHT CHANGE	☐	FLUE-LIKE	☐
CHILLS	☐	BRAIN FOG	☐

Pain & Inflammation

JOINT PAIN	☐	JOINT SWELLING	☐
STIFFNESS	☐	MUSCLE ACHES	☐
WEAKNESS	☐	BACK PAIN	☐
NERVE PAIN	☐	MIGRAINES	☐

Thyroid-like

TREMORS	☐	HEART PALPITATIONS	☐
HEAT/COLD SENSITITVITY	☐	WEIGHT SHIFT	☐
CHILLS	☐	NECK PAIN	☐

Skin, Hair & Nails

RASH	☐	REDNESS/FLUSHING	☐
HIVES	☐	SENSITITIY TO SUN	☐
ITCHING	☐	BRITTLE NAILS	☐
HAIR LOSS	☐	DRY SKIN	☐

Respiratory

CHEST PAIN	☐	CHRONIC COUGH	☐
SHORTNESS OF BREATH	☐		

Kidneys

FOAMY URINE	☐	SWELLING IN LEGS / ANKLES	☐
DARK URINE	☐	BLOODY URINE	☐

Digestive / GI

NAUSEA	☐	STOMACH PAINS	☐
VOMITING	☐	FOOD REACTIONS	☐
DIARRHEA	☐	APPETITE LOSS	☐
CONSTIPATION	☐	BLOATING	☐

Vascular

NUMB FINGERS/TOES	☐	RAYNAUD'S COLOR CHANGES	☐

DAILY SYMPTOM TRACKER

Date:

Stress Level

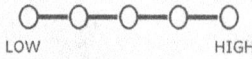

LOW   HIGH

Today's Water Intake

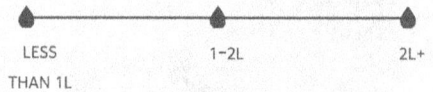

LESS THAN 1L   1-2L   2L+

Pain's Impact On Today's Function

Today pain affected my ability to:

DRIVE ☐   WORK ☐   SOCIALIZE ☐

COOK ☐   LIFT/CARRY ☐   LEAVE THE HOUSE ☐

WALK ☐   CARE FOR SELF ☐   SIT/LAY DOWN ☐

Food & Immune Response

DID YOU EAT ANYTHING NEW TODAY?

YES ☐   NO ☐

Impact On Symptoms

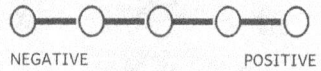

NEGATIVE   POSITIVE

Notes

_____

_____

_____

_____

_____

_____

Symptom Changes Throughout The Day

CONSISTENT ☐   WORSE AT NIGHT ☐

COMES IN WAVES ☐   PAIN FLARE ☐

WORSE IN MORNING ☐

Notes

_____

_____

_____

_____

_____

_____

_____

_____

_____

Activity Overview

REST DAY ☐   LIGHT MOVEMENT ☐

MODERATE ACTIVITY ☐   HEAVY ACTIVITY ☐

Effect On Pain

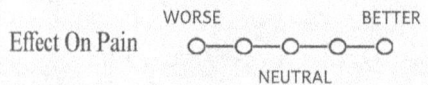

WORSE   BETTER

NEUTRAL

DAILY SYMPTOM TRACKER

Date:

Sleep QUALITY (1-10) _____ LENGTH _____

Weather
HOT ☐ DRY ☐ HUMID ☐
RAIN ☐ STORM ☐ COLD ☐

Flare Status
SUDDEN ☐ TRIGGERED ☐
SLOW BUILDING ☐ RANDOM ☐

NO FLARE ○ ○ ○ ○ ○ SEVERE FLAIR
MILD   MODERATE

SUSPECTED TRIGGER _____

Today's Symptoms

	LOW	HIGH
FEVER	O—O—O—O—O	
FATIGUE	O—O—O—O—O	

Systemic
DIZZINESS	☐	NIGHT SWEATS	☐
WEIGHT CHANGE	☐	FLUE-LIKE	☐
CHILLS	☐	BRAIN FOG	☐

Pain & Inflammation
JOINT PAIN	☐	JOINT SWELLING	☐
STIFFNESS	☐	MUSCLE ACHES	☐
WEAKNESS	☐	BACK PAIN	☐
NERVE PAIN	☐	MIGRAINES	☐

Thyroid-like
TREMORS	☐	HEART PALPITATIONS	☐
HEAT/COLD SENSITITVITY	☐	WEIGHT SHIFT	☐
CHILLS	☐	NECK PAIN	☐

Skin, Hair & Nails
RASH	☐	REDNESS/FLUSHING	☐
HIVES	☐	SENSITITY TO SUN	☐
ITCHING	☐	BRITTLE NAILS	☐
HAIR LOSS	☐	DRY SKIN	☐

Respiratory
CHEST PAIN	☐	CHRONIC COUGH	☐
SHORTNESS OF BREATH	☐		

Kidneys
FOAMY URINE	☐	SWELLING IN LEGS / ANKLES	☐
DARK URINE	☐	BLOODY URINE	☐

Digestive / GI
NAUSEA	☐	STOMACH PAINS	☐
VOMITING	☐	FOOD REACTIONS	☐
DIARRHEA	☐	APPETITE LOSS	☐
CONSTIPATION	☐	BLOATING	☐

Vascular
NUMB FINGERS/TOES	☐	RAYNAUD'S COLOR CHANGES	☐

DAILY SYMPTOM TRACKER

Date:

Stress Level O—O—O—O—O

LOW   HIGH

Pain's Impact On Today's Function
Today pain affected my ability to:

DRIVE ☐   WORK ☐   SOCIALIZE ☐

COOK ☐   LIFT/CARRY ☐   LEAVE THE HOUSE ☐

WALK ☐   CARE FOR SELF ☐   SIT/LAY DOWN ☐

Symptom Changes Throughout The Day

CONSISTENT ☐   WORSE AT NIGHT ☐

COMES IN WAVES ☐   PAIN FLARE ☐

WORSE IN MORNING ☐

Notes

_____

_____

_____

_____

_____

_____

_____

_____

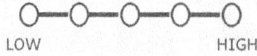

Today's Water Intake

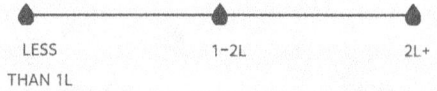

O———————O———————O

LESS THAN 1L   1–2L   2L+

Food & Immune Response

DID YOU EAT ANYTHING NEW TODAY?

YES ☐   NO ☐

Impact On Symptoms

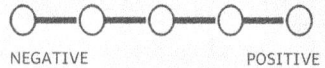

O—O—O—O—O

NEGATIVE   POSITIVE

Notes

_____

_____

_____

_____

_____

_____

Activity Overview

REST DAY ☐   LIGHT MOVEMENT ☐

MODERATE ACTIVITY ☐   HEAVY ACTIVITY ☐

           WORSE   BETTER

Effect On Pain   O—O—O—O—O

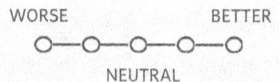

               NEUTRAL

DAILY SYMPTOM TRACKER

Date:

Sleep QUALITY (1-10) _____ LENGTH _____

Flare Status SUDDEN ☐ TRIGGERED ☐ SLOW BUILDING ☐ RANDOM ☐

NO FLARE ○ ○ ○ ○ ○ SEVERE FLAIR
MILD   MODERATE

Weather HOT ☐ DRY ☐ HUMID ☐ RAIN ☐ STORM ☐ COLD ☐

SUSPECTED TRIGGER _____

Today's Symptoms

Systemic

DIZZINESS	☐	NIGHT SWEATS	☐
WEIGHT CHANGE	☐	FLUE-LIKE	☐
CHILLS	☐	BRAIN FOG	☐

LOW — HIGH
FEVER   ○—○—○—○—○
FATIGUE ○—○—○—○—○

Pain & Inflammation

JOINT PAIN	☐	JOINT SWELLING	☐
STIFFNESS	☐	MUSCLE ACHES	☐
WEAKNESS	☐	BACK PAIN	☐
NERVE PAIN	☐	MIGRAINES	☐

Thyroid-like

TREMORS	☐	HEART PALPITATIONS	☐
HEAT/COLD SENSITITVITY	☐	WEIGHT SHIFT	☐
CHILLS	☐	NECK PAIN	☐

Skin, Hair & Nails

RASH	☐	REDNESS/FLUSHING	☐
HIVES	☐	SENSITITY TO SUN	☐
ITCHING	☐	BRITTLE NAILS	☐
HAIR LOSS	☐	DRY SKIN	☐

Respiratory

CHEST PAIN	☐	CHRONIC COUGH	☐
SHORTNESS OF BREATH	☐		

Kidneys

FOAMY URINE	☐	SWELLING IN LEGS / ANKLES	☐
DARK URINE	☐	BLOODY URINE	☐

Digestive / GI

NAUSEA	☐	STOMACH PAINS	☐
VOMITING	☐	FOOD REACTIONS	☐
DIARRHEA	☐	APPETITE LOSS	☐
CONSTIPATION	☐	BLOATING	☐

Vascular

NUMB FINGERS/TOES	☐	RAYNAUD'S COLOR CHANGES	☐

DAILY SYMPTOM TRACKER

Date:

Stress Level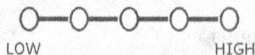
LOW   HIGH

Today's Water Intake

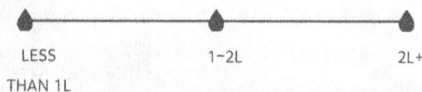

LESS   1–2L   2L+
THAN 1L

Pain's Impact On Today's Function
Today pain affected my ability to:

DRIVE ☐   WORK ☐   SOCIALIZE ☐

COOK ☐   LIFT/CARRY ☐   LEAVE THE HOUSE ☐

WALK ☐   CARE FOR SELF ☐   SIT/LAY DOWN ☐

Food & Immune Response

DID YOU EAT ANYTHING NEW TODAY?

YES ☐   NO ☐

Impact On Symptoms

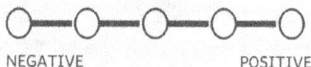

NEGATIVE   POSITIVE

Notes

_____

_____

_____

_____

_____

_____

Symptom Changes Throughout The Day

CONSISTENT ☐   WORSE AT NIGHT ☐

COMES IN WAVES ☐   PAIN FLARE ☐

WORSE IN MORNING ☐

Notes

_____

_____

_____

_____

_____

_____

_____

Activity Overview

REST DAY ☐   LIGHT MOVEMENT ☐

MODERATE ACTIVITY ☐   HEAVY ACTIVITY ☐

WORSE   BETTER

Effect On Pain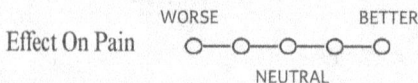

NEUTRAL

DAILY SYMPTOM TRACKER

Date:

Sleep
QUALITY (1-10) _____ LENGTH _____

Weather
HOT ☐ DRY ☐ HUMID ☐
RAIN ☐ STORM ☐ COLD ☐

Flare Status
SUDDEN ☐ TRIGGERED ☐
SLOW BUILDING ☐ RANDOM ☐

NO FLARE ○——○——○——○——○ SEVERE FLAIR
    MILD   MODERATE

SUSPECTED TRIGGER _____

Today's Symptoms

	LOW	HIGH
FEVER	○—○—○—○—○	
FATIGUE	○—○—○—○—○	

Systemic

DIZZINESS	☐	NIGHT SWEATS	☐
WEIGHT CHANGE	☐	FLUE-LIKE	☐
CHILLS	☐	BRAIN FOG	☐

Pain & Inflammation

JOINT PAIN	☐	JOINT SWELLING	☐
STIFFNESS	☐	MUSCLE ACHES	☐
WEAKNESS	☐	BACK PAIN	☐
NERVE PAIN	☐	MIGRAINES	☐

Thyroid-like

TREMORS	☐	HEART PALPITATIONS	☐
HEAT/COLD SENSITITVITY	☐	WEIGHT SHIFT	☐
CHILLS	☐	NECK PAIN	☐

Skin, Hair & Nails

RASH	☐	REDNESS/FLUSHING	☐
HIVES	☐	SENSITITITY TO SUN	☐
ITCHING	☐	BRITTLE NAILS	☐
HAIR LOSS	☐	DRY SKIN	☐

Respiratory

CHEST PAIN	☐	CHRONIC COUGH	☐
SHORTNESS OF BREATH	☐		

Kidneys

FOAMY URINE	☐	SWELLING IN LEGS / ANKLES	☐
DARK URINE	☐	BLOODY URINE	☐

Digestive / GI

NAUSEA	☐	STOMACH PAINS	☐
VOMITING	☐	FOOD REACTIONS	☐
DIARRHEA	☐	APPETITE LOSS	☐
CONSTIPATION	☐	BLOATING	☐

Vascular

NUMB FINGERS/TOES	☐	RAYNAUD'S COLOR CHANGES	☐

DAILY SYMPTOM TRACKER

Date:

Stress Level

O—O—O—O—O

LOW   HIGH

Pain's Impact On Today's Function
Today pain affected my ability to:

DRIVE ☐   WORK ☐   SOCIALIZE ☐

COOK ☐   LIFT/CARRY ☐   LEAVE THE HOUSE ☐

WALK ☐   CARE FOR SELF ☐   SIT/LAY DOWN ☐

Symptom Changes Throughout The Day

CONSISTENT ☐   WORSE AT NIGHT ☐

COMES IN WAVES ☐   PAIN FLARE ☐

WORSE IN MORNING ☐

Notes

_____

_____

_____

_____

_____

_____

_____

_____

Today's Water Intake

●————————●————————●

LESS THAN 1L   1–2L   2L+

Food & Immune Response

DID YOU EAT ANYTHING NEW TODAY?

YES ☐   NO ☐

Impact On Symptoms

O—O—O—O—O

NEGATIVE   POSITIVE

Notes

_____

_____

_____

_____

_____

_____

Activity Overview

REST DAY ☐   LIGHT MOVEMENT ☐

MODERATE ACTIVITY ☐   HEAVY ACTIVITY ☐

Effect On Pain

WORSE   BETTER

O—O—O—O—O

NEUTRAL

DAILY SYMPTOM TRACKER

Date:

Sleep
QUALITY (1-10) _____ LENGTH _____

Weather
HOT ☐ DRY ☐ HUMID ☐
RAIN ☐ STORM ☐ COLD ☐

Flare Status
SUDDEN ☐ TRIGGERED ☐
SLOW BUILDING ☐ RANDOM ☐

NO FLARE ○ ○ ○ ○ ○ SEVERE FLAIR
MILD MODERATE

SUSPECTED TRIGGER _____

Today's Symptoms

	LOW	HIGH
FEVER	○—○—○—○—○	
FATIGUE	○—○—○—○—○	

Systemic

DIZZINESS ☐ NIGHT SWEATS ☐
WEIGHT CHANGE ☐ FLUE-LIKE ☐
CHILLS ☐ BRAIN FOG ☐

Pain & Inflammation

JOINT PAIN ☐ JOINT SWELLING ☐
STIFFNESS ☐ MUSCLE ACHES ☐
WEAKNESS ☐ BACK PAIN ☐
NERVE PAIN ☐ MIGRAINES ☐

Thyroid-like

TREMORS ☐ HEART PALPITATIONS ☐
HEAT/COLD SENSITITVITY ☐ WEIGHT SHIFT ☐
CHILLS ☐ NECK PAIN ☐

Skin, Hair & Nails

RASH ☐ REDNESS/FLUSHING ☐
HIVES ☐ SENSITITY TO SUN ☐
ITCHING ☐ BRITTLE NAILS ☐
HAIR LOSS ☐ DRY SKIN ☐

Respiratory

CHEST PAIN ☐ CHRONIC COUGH ☐
SHORTNESS OF BREATH ☐

Kidneys

FOAMY URINE ☐ SWELLING IN LEGS / ANKLES ☐
DARK URINE ☐ BLOODY URINE ☐

Digestive / GI

NAUSEA ☐ STOMACH PAINS ☐
VOMITING ☐ FOOD REACTIONS ☐
DIARRHEA ☐ APPETITE LOSS ☐
CONSTIPATION ☐ BLOATING ☐

Vascular

NUMB FINGERS/TOES ☐ RAYNAUD'S COLOR CHANGES ☐

DAILY SYMPTOM TRACKER

Date: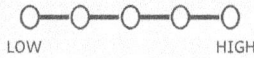

Stress Level
LOW   HIGH

Today's Water Intake
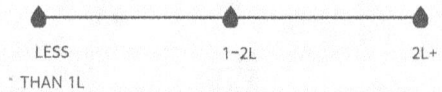

LESS THAN 1L   1-2L   2L+

Pain's Impact On Today's Function
Today pain affected my ability to:

DRIVE ☐   WORK ☐   SOCIALIZE ☐

COOK ☐   LIFT/CARRY ☐   LEAVE THE HOUSE ☐

WALK ☐   CARE FOR SELF ☐   SIT/LAY DOWN ☐

Food & Immune Response
DID YOU EAT ANYTHING NEW TODAY?

YES ☐   NO ☐

Impact On Symptoms
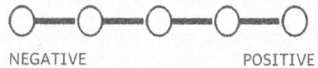

NEGATIVE   POSITIVE

Notes
_____
_____
_____
_____
_____
_____

Symptom Changes Throughout The Day

CONSISTENT ☐   WORSE AT NIGHT ☐

COMES IN WAVES ☐   PAIN FLARE ☐

WORSE IN MORNING ☐

Notes
_____
_____
_____
_____
_____
_____
_____
_____
_____
_____

Activity Overview

REST DAY ☐   LIGHT MOVEMENT ☐

MODERATE ACTIVITY ☐   HEAVY ACTIVITY ☐

Effect On Pain
WORSE   BETTER

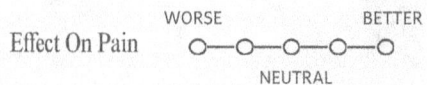

NEUTRAL

DAILY SYMPTOM TRACKER

Date:

Sleep
QUALITY (1-10) _____ LENGTH _____

Weather
HOT ☐   DRY ☐   HUMID ☐
RAIN ☐   STORM ☐   COLD ☐

Flare Status
SUDDEN ☐   TRIGGERED ☐
SLOW BUILDING ☐   RANDOM ☐

NO FLARE ○——○——○——○——○ SEVERE FLAIR
MILD   MODERATE

SUSPECTED TRIGGER _____

Today's Symptoms

	LOW	HIGH
FEVER	○—○—○—○—○	
FATIGUE	○—○—○—○—○	

Systemic
DIZZINESS	☐	NIGHT SWEATS	☐
WEIGHT CHANGE	☐	FLUE-LIKE	☐
CHILLS	☐	BRAIN FOG	☐

Pain & Inflammation
JOINT PAIN	☐	JOINT SWELLING	☐
STIFFNESS	☐	MUSCLE ACHES	☐
WEAKNESS	☐	BACK PAIN	☐
NERVE PAIN	☐	MIGRAINES	☐

Thyroid-like
TREMORS	☐	HEART PALPITATIONS	☐
HEAT/COLD SENSITITVITY	☐	WEIGHT SHIFT	☐
CHILLS	☐	NECK PAIN	☐

Skin, Hair & Nails
RASH	☐	REDNESS/FLUSHING	☐
HIVES	☐	SENSITITITY TO SUN	☐
ITCHING	☐	BRITTLE NAILS	☐
HAIR LOSS	☐	DRY SKIN	☐

Respiratory
CHEST PAIN	☐	CHRONIC COUGH	☐
SHORTNESS OF BREATH	☐		

Kidneys
FOAMY URINE	☐	SWELLING IN LEGS / ANKLES	☐
DARK URINE	☐	BLOODY URINE	☐

Digestive / GI
NAUSEA	☐	STOMACH PAINS	☐
VOMITING	☐	FOOD REACTIONS	☐
DIARRHEA	☐	APPETITE LOSS	☐
CONSTIPATION	☐	BLOATING	☐

Vascular
NUMB FINGERS/TOES	☐	RAYNAUD'S COLOR CHANGES	☐

DAILY SYMPTOM TRACKER

Date:

Stress Level O—O—O—O—O
LOW   HIGH

Today's Water Intake

LESS THAN 1L   1–2L   2L+

Pain's Impact On Today's Function
Today pain affected my ability to:

DRIVE ☐   WORK ☐   SOCIALIZE ☐

COOK ☐   LIFT/CARRY ☐   LEAVE THE HOUSE ☐

WALK ☐   CARE FOR SELF ☐ SIT/LAY DOWN ☐

Food & Immune Response

DID YOU EAT ANYTHING NEW TODAY?

YES ☐   NO ☐

Impact On Symptoms

O—O—O—O—O
NEGATIVE   POSITIVE

Notes

_____
_____
_____
_____
_____
_____

Symptom Changes Throughout The Day

CONSISTENT ☐   WORSE AT NIGHT ☐

COMES IN WAVES ☐   PAIN FLARE ☐

WORSE IN MORNING ☐

Notes

_____
_____
_____
_____
_____
_____
_____
_____

Activity Overview

REST DAY ☐   LIGHT MOVEMENT ☐

MODERATE ACTIVITY ☐   HEAVY ACTIVITY ☐

Effect On Pain   WORSE   BETTER
                      O—O—O—O—O
                        NEUTRAL

IMPORTANT NOTES

_____
_____
_____
_____
_____
_____
_____
_____
_____
_____
_____
_____
_____
_____
_____
_____
_____
_____
_____
_____

WEEKLY SUMMARY

Week Of:

Sleep	Overall Feelings
QUALITY (1-10) _____	MOOD (1-10) _____ MENTAL CLARITY (1-10) _____ ENERGY (1-10) _____ IMPACT FROM WEATHER (1-10)_____

Autoimmune Flare Snapshot

This week:

I EXPERIENCED UNUSUAL FATIGUE	NOT AT ALL ☐	SEVERAL TIMES ☐	OFTEN ☐	CONSTANT ☐
MY PAIN WAS	LOW ☐	MILD ☐	WORSE ☐	CONSTANT ☐
I HAD MORNING STIFFNESS	NOT AT ALL ☐	30 MINUTES ☐	30-60 ☐	OVER 60 ☐
MY SYMPTOMS WORSENED WITH ACTIVITY	NOT AT ALL ☐	SEVERAL TIMES ☐	OFTEN ☐	CONSTANT ☐
MY SYMPTOMS WORSENED WITH REST	NOT AT ALL ☐	SEVERAL TIMES ☐	OFTEN ☐	CONSTANT ☐
I HAD FLU-LIKE SENSATIONS	NOT AT ALL ☐	SEVERAL TIMES ☐	OFTEN ☐	CONSTANT ☐

FATIGUE & ENERGY CHECK-IN

This week made feel:

FEELING "POISONED" OR SICK	NOT AT ALL ☐	SEVERAL TIMES ☐	OFTEN ☐	CONSTANT ☐
EXHAUSTION AFTER SMALL TASKS	NOT AT ALL ☐	SEVERAL TIMES ☐	OFTEN ☐	CONSTANT ☐
FEELING TIRED EVEN AFTER RESTING	NOT AT ALL ☐	SEVERAL TIMES ☐	OFTEN ☐	CONSTANT ☐
MUSCLES FEELING WEAK OR "HEAVY"	NOT AT ALL ☐	SEVERAL TIMES ☐	OFTEN ☐	CONSTANT ☐
NEEDING NAPS TO FUNCTION	NOT AT ALL ☐	SEVERAL TIMES ☐	OFTEN ☐	CONSTANT ☐
BRAIN FOG INTERFERING WITH THINKING	NOT AT ALL ☐	SEVERAL TIMES ☐	OFTEN ☐	CONSTANT ☐

MOBILITY CHECK-IN

During this week, how often did you experience:

STIFFNESS IN THE MORNING	NOT AT ALL ☐	SEVERAL TIMES ☐	OFTEN ☐	CONSTANT ☐
DIFFICULTY GETTING OUT OF BED	NOT AT ALL ☐	SEVERAL TIMES ☐	OFTEN ☐	CONSTANT ☐
REDUCED RANGE OF MOTION	NOT AT ALL ☐	SEVERAL TIMES ☐	OFTEN ☐	CONSTANT ☐
TROUBLE GRIPPING OR LIFTING	NOT AT ALL ☐	SEVERAL TIMES ☐	OFTEN ☐	CONSTANT ☐
SLOWER WALKING SPEED	NOT AT ALL ☐	SEVERAL TIMES ☐	OFTEN ☐	CONSTANT ☐
FEELING UNSTABLE OR WEAK	NOT AT ALL ☐	SEVERAL TIMES ☐	OFTEN ☐	CONSTANT ☐
NEEDED MOBILITY AIDS	NOT AT ALL ☐	SEVERAL TIMES ☐	OFTEN ☐	CONSTANT ☐

WEEKLY SUMMARY

Week Of:

Sleep	Overall Feelings
QUALITY (1–10) _____	MOOD (1–10) _____ MENTAL CLARITY (1–10) _____
	ENERGY (1–10) _____ IMPACT FROM WEATHER (1–10) _____

RED FLAG CHECK-IN

During this week, did you notice:

NEW NUMBNESS	NOT AT ALL ☐ SEVERAL TIMES ☐	OFTEN ☐	CONSTANT ☐
NEW WEAKNESS	NOT AT ALL ☐ SEVERAL TIMES ☐	OFTEN ☐	CONSTANT ☐
PAIN THAT WOKE ME FROM SLEEP	NOT AT ALL ☐ SEVERAL TIMES ☐	OFTEN ☐	CONSTANT ☐
LOSS OF BLADDER/BOWEL CONTROL	NOT AT ALL ☐ SEVERAL TIMES ☐	OFTEN ☐	CONSTANT ☐
SUDDEN SEVERE PAIN	NOT AT ALL ☐ SEVERAL TIMES ☐	OFTEN ☐	CONSTANT ☐
NEW SWELLING/REDNESS	NOT AT ALL ☐ SEVERAL TIMES ☐	OFTEN ☐	CONSTANT ☐

IT IS ESSENTIAL TO BRING THESE RESULTS UP WITH YOUR HEALTHCARE PROVIDER AS SOON AS POSSIBLE.

FLARE PATTERN CHECK-IN

During this week, I had flares that felt:

SUDDEN	NOT AT ALL ☐	SEVERAL TIMES ☐	OFTEN ☐
SLOW–BUILDING	NOT AT ALL ☐	SEVERAL TIMES ☐	OFTEN ☐
TRIGGERED	NOT AT ALL ☐	SEVERAL TIMES ☐	OFTEN ☐
RANDOM	NOT AT ALL ☐	SEVERAL TIMES ☐	OFTEN ☐
WORSE THAN USUAL	NOT AT ALL ☐	SEVERAL TIMES ☐	OFTEN ☐
UNUSUAL COMPARED TO TYPICAL FLARES	NOT AT ALL ☐	SEVERAL TIMES ☐	OFTEN ☐

DURATION OF FLARES _____

Notes

_____

_____

_____

_____

WEEKLY SUMMARY
PATTERNS & NOTES

Week Of:

_____

Patterns / Similarities On Good Days

- ○ _____
- ○ _____
- ○ _____
- ○ _____
- ○ _____

Patterns / Similarities On Bad Days

- ○ _____
- ○ _____
- ○ _____
- ○ _____
- ○ _____

Things That Improved Symptoms

- ○ _____
- ○ _____
- ○ _____
- ○ _____
- ○ _____

WEEKLY SUMMARY
PATTERNS & NOTES

Week Of:

Most Common Symptoms

○ _____
○ _____
○ _____
○ _____
○ _____

Most Common Triggers

○ _____
○ _____
○ _____
○ _____
○ _____

Symptom Timing Patterns

When do your symptoms tend to be at their worst?

MORNING ☐   AFTER MEALS ☐
AFTERNOON ☐   AFTER PHYSICAL ACTIVITY ☐
EVENING ☐   HORMONE FLUCTUATIONS ☐
NIGHT ☐   DURING STRESS ☐
UPON WAKING ☐   DURING WEATHER CHANGES ☐

NOTES

_____
_____
_____
_____
_____
_____
_____
_____
_____
_____
_____
_____
_____
_____

Overall Effectiveness Of Treatment This Week

○──────○──────○──────○──────○
LOW   HIGH

Overall Stress This Week

○──────○──────○──────○──────○
LOW   HIGH

Overall Sleep This Week

○──────○──────○──────○──────○
LOW   HIGH

SUMMARY PATTERNS
PATTERNS & NOTES

Most Common Symptoms *(physical, psychological, etc.)*

SYMPTOM	TRIGGER	WHAT HAPPENED (RESULT)	DURATION

Most Effective Treatments *(physical therapy, medication, supplements)*

SYMPTOM	TREATMENT	EFFECTIVENESS (1-10)	LONG TERM IMPROVEMENT (Y/N)

SUMMARY PATTERNS
PATTERNS & NOTES

Most Common Symptoms   *(physical, psychological, etc.)*

SYMPTOM	TRIGGER	WHAT HAPPENED (RESULT)	DURATION

Most Effective Treatments   *(physical therapy, medication, supplements)*

SYMPTOM	TREATMENT	EFFECTIVENESS (1-10)	LONG TERM IMPROVEMENT (Y/N)

SELF-DIAGNOSTIC ASSISTANT

Primary Sorting Questions

Circle yes or no. Follow the arrows.

1. DO YOUR SYMPTOMS COME IN "FLARES" (BAD DAYS) AND "REMISSIONS"

   (BETTER DAYS)?

   o YES → GO TO #2

   o NO → GO TO #3

2. DO FLARES LAST LONGER THAN 24-48 HOURS?

   o YES → YOU MAY LEAN INFLAMMATORY

   o NO → YOU MAY LEAN REACTIVE/SENSITIVITY-BASED

3. DO YOU EXPERIENCE SYMPTOMS IN MULTIPLE BODY SYSTEMS AT THE SAME

   TIME?

4. (E.G., SKIN + JOINTS, OR FATIGUE + DIGESTION, OR MOOD + PAIN)

   o YES → SYSTEMIC OR CONNECTIVE TISSUE CLUSTER

   o NO → LOCALIZED CLUSTER

5. DO SYMPTOMS FOLLOW PREDICTABLE TRIGGERS (WEATHER, STRESS, FOODS,

   HORMONES, INFECTION)?

   o YES → TRIGGER-SENSITIVE CLUSTER

   o NO → CHECK CENTRAL/MIXED CLUSTER

SELF-DIAGNOSTIC ASSISTANT

Check the statements that apply. Your cluster is whichever group has the most checkmarks. These clusters represent symptom patterns, not diagnoses.

Cluster A — Inflammatory Body Cluster

(Classic autoimmune flare pattern)

YOU MAY RELATE IF YOU EXPERIENCE:
- MORNING STIFFNESS OR PAIN
- HEAT, SWELLING, REDNESS IN JOINTS
- DEEP FATIGUE THAT FEELS "IN YOUR BONES"
- PAIN THAT IMPROVES SLOWLY THROUGHOUT THE DAY
- WEATHER OR TEMPERATURE SENSITIVITY
- FLARES AFTER OVEREXERTION

EXAMPLES OF CONDITIONS DOCTORS CONSIDER UNDER THIS PATTERN:

RHEUMATOID-TYPE INFLAMMATION, PSORIATIC-TYPE PROCESSES, ANKYLOSING-TYPE PATTERNS.

(NOT DIAGNOSING — JUST EXPLAINING THE PATTERN.

Cluster B — Autoimmune Skin + Barrier Cluster

(Immune issues in skin, hair, nails, or mucous membranes)

YOU MAY RELATE IF YOU NOTICE:
- RASHES, HIVES, OR UNEXPLAINED REDNESS
- FLAKY, ITCHY, OR BURNING PATCHES
- FREQUENT MOUTH ULCERS
- HAIR SHEDDING OR THINNING
- NAIL RIDGING, PITTING, OR WEAKNESS
- REACTIONS TO PRODUCTS, FRAGRANCES, STRESS, OR ILLNESS

THIS CLUSTER OFTEN OVERLAPS WITH ECZEMA-LIKE, PSORIASIS-LIKE, OR ALOPECIA-TYPE PATTERNS.

Cluster C — Digestive + Immune Reactivity Cluster

(Immune activation connected to the gut)

PATTERNS MAY INCLUDE:
- BLOATING, ABDOMINAL DISCOMFORT
- FOOD-TRIGGERED SYMPTOMS
- BRAIN FOG AFTER MEALS
- JOINT OR SKIN FLARES CONNECTED TO DIGESTION
- CONSTIPATION/DIARRHEA CYCLING
- FEELING INFLAMED AFTER CERTAIN FOODS

PEOPLE IN THIS CLUSTER OFTEN NOTE THAT IMMUNE SYMPTOMS AND GUT SYMPTOMS MOVE TOGETHER.

SELF-DIAGNOSTIC ASSISTANT

Check the statements that apply. Your cluster is whichever group has the most checkmarks. These clusters represent symptom patterns, not diagnoses.

Cluster D — Systemic + Connective Tissue Cluster

(Body-wide patterns affecting multiple systems)

YOU MAY RELATE IF YOU NOTICE:
- FATIGUE + JOINT PAIN + DRYNESS (EYES, MOUTH)
- DIZZINESS OR "INTERNAL WEAKNESS"
- SKIN SENSITIVITY
- MUSCLE ACHES OR WEAKNESS
- UNEXPLAINED ORGAN INVOLVEMENT (THYROID, LUNGS, ETC.)
- NUMBNESS OR TINGLING WITHOUT CLEAR CAUSE

THIS CLUSTER TENDS TO FEEL "FULL-BODY," NOT JUST ONE LOCATION.

Cluster E — Mixed Autoimmune-Like Cluster

If your symptoms jump across categories or change frequently, you may fall here.

THIS CLUSTER FITS PEOPLE WHO SAY:
- "I HAVE INFLAMMATION SOMETIMES, SENSITIVITIES SOMETIMES, FATIGUE ALWAYS, AND I CAN'T FIGURE OUT THE PATTERN."
- "EVERYTHING SEEMS CONNECTED EVEN THOUGH I CAN'T PROVE IT."

THIS IS VERY COMMON EARLY IN AUTOIMMUNE INVESTIGATION.

SELF-DIAGNOSTIC ASSISTANT
PATTERN SUMMARY PAGE

I seem to fall mostly into Cluster: _____

Secondary cluster (if any): _____

My flares look like:

_____

_____

_____

Triggers I've noticed:

_____

_____

_____

_____

Systems involved:

_____

_____

_____

_____

Frequency + severity pattern:

_____

_____

_____

_____

SELF-DIAGNOSTIC ASSISTANT
SPEAKING WITH YOUR DOCTOR

Short Example:

"I've been tracking my symptoms for several weeks using this journal, and I'm noticing some repeating patterns. They aren't random—they follow certain triggers, flare in certain ways, and often involve multiple systems. I'm not trying to diagnose myself, but these patterns seem important, so I wanted to show you the logs I collected. Could we look at these together and discuss what might be worth testing or exploring next?"

Now the specific add-ons for each cluster:

Cluster A – Inflammatory Body Add-On

"My symptoms worsen in the morning and improve later in the day, and I have flare days that last longer than 24 hours."

Cluster B – Skin/Barrier Add-On

"I'm getting recurring skin/hair/nail symptoms that seem tied to stress, foods, or immune activity."

Cluster C – Digestive Reactivity Add-On

"My immune-type symptoms often appear after meals or digestive flare-ups."

Cluster D – Systemic/Add-On

"Multiple systems are involved, including fatigue, joints, and dryness, and the symptoms seem connected."

Cluster E – Mixed/Unclear Add-On

"My symptoms move across categories, and I can't find one source — but the pattern itself is consistent."

NOTES FROM APPOINTMENT

DATE

DOCTOR'S NAME

SATISFACTION WITH APPOINTMENT ☹ ☹ ☺ ☺ ☺

POINTS FROM TODAY'S APPOINTMENT

1.

2.

3.

THOUGHTS & REFLECTIONS

LAB & TEST RESULTS
PATTERNS & NOTES

Date:

TEST NAME

LOCATION

WHAT WAS
BEING
INVESTIGATED

RESULTS

NOTES

IMPORTANT NOTES

NEW TREATMENT
HEALING YOURSELF

Keeping a clear record of what you try — and how it affects you — is one of the most powerful tools for understanding your health. This page helps you track medications, supplements, therapies, or lifestyle changes in one place, making it easier to see patterns and share accurate information with your healthcare provider.

This New Treatment Is

MEDICATION ☐   SUPPLEMENT ☐   PHYSICAL THERAPY ☐   OTHER: ☐

This Was

PRESCRIBED ☐   RECOMMENDED ☐

START DATE _____

Schedule

DOSAGE _____

FREQUENCY _____

Expected Reactions

○ _____
○ _____
○ _____
○ _____
○ _____

Unexpected Side Effects

○ _____
○ _____
○ _____
○ _____
○ _____

Positive Impact On Daily Function

ABILITY TO WORK (1–10)   _____
SOCIAL INTERACTIONS (1–10)   _____
CONCENTRATION (1–10)   _____
ENERGY / MOTIVATION (1–10)   _____
PHYSICAL ACTIVITY (1–10)   _____
WELLNESS (1–10)   _____

Treatment Effectiveness

○────○────○────○────○
LOW   HIGH

Treatment Impact

○────○────○────○────○
NEGATIVE   POSITIVE

Going Forward: CHANGE DOSAGE/ FREQUENCY ☐   TERMINATE USE ☐   CONTINUE USE ☐

NOTES FROM APPOINTMENT

DATE

DOCTOR'S NAME

SATISFACTION WITH APPOINTMENT ☹ ☹ 😐 🙂 😊

POINTS FROM TODAY'S APPOINTMENT

1.

2.

3.

THOUGHTS & REFLECTIONS

LAB & TEST RESULTS
PATTERNS & NOTES

Date:

TEST NAME

LOCATION

WHAT WAS
BEING
INVESTIGATED

RESULTS

NOTES

IMPORTANT NOTES

NEW TREATMENT
HEALING YOURSELF

Keeping a clear record of what you try — and how it affects you — is one of the most powerful tools for understanding your health. This page helps you track medications, supplements, therapies, or lifestyle changes in one place, making it easier to see patterns and share accurate information with your healthcare provider.

This New Treatment Is

MEDICATION ☐   SUPPLEMENT ☐   PHYSICAL THERAPY ☐   OTHER: ☐

This Was

PRESCRIBED ☐   RECOMMENDED ☐

START DATE _____

Schedule

DOSAGE _____

FREQUENCY _____

Expected Reactions

○ _____
○ _____
○ _____
○ _____
○ _____

Unexpected Side Effects

○ _____
○ _____
○ _____
○ _____
○ _____

Positive Impact On Daily Function

ABILITY TO WORK (1–10) _____
SOCIAL INTERACTIONS (1–10) _____
CONCENTRATION (1–10) _____
ENERGY / MOTIVATION (1–10) _____
PHYSICAL ACTIVITY (1–10) _____
WELLNESS (1–10) _____

Treatment Effectiveness

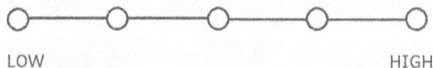

○———○———○———○———○
LOW   HIGH

Treatment Impact

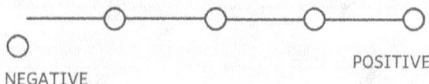

○———○———○———○
NEGATIVE   POSITIVE

Going Forward: CHANGE DOSAGE/ FREQUENCY ☐   TERMINATE USE ☐   CONTINUE USE ☐

NOTES FROM APPOINTMENT

DATE

DOCTOR'S NAME

SATISFACTION WITH APPOINTMENT

POINTS FROM TODAY'S APPOINTMENT

1.

2.

3.

THOUGHTS & REFLECTIONS

LAB & TEST RESULTS
PATTERNS & NOTES

Date:

TEST NAME

LOCATION

WHAT WAS
BEING
INVESTIGATED

RESULTS

NOTES

IMPORTANT NOTES

NEW TREATMENT
HEALING YOURSELF

Keeping a clear record of what you try — and how it affects you — is one of the most powerful tools for understanding your health. This page helps you track medications, supplements, therapies, or lifestyle changes in one place, making it easier to see patterns and share accurate information with your healthcare provider.

This New Treatment Is

MEDICATION ☐   SUPPLEMENT ☐   PHYSICAL THERAPY ☐   OTHER: ☐

This Was

PRESCRIBED ☐   RECOMMENDED ☐

START DATE _____

Schedule

DOSAGE _____

FREQUENCY _____

Expected Reactions

○ _____
○ _____
○ _____
○ _____
○ _____

Unexpected Side Effects

○ _____
○ _____
○ _____
○ _____
○ _____

Positive Impact On Daily Function

ABILITY TO WORK (1–10) _____
SOCIAL INTERACTIONS (1–10) _____
CONCENTRATION (1–10) _____
ENERGY / MOTIVATION (1–10) _____
PHYSICAL ACTIVITY (1–10) _____
WELLNESS (1–10) _____

Treatment Effectiveness

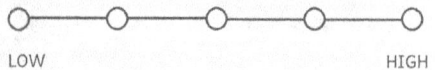

○——○——○——○——○
LOW   HIGH

Treatment Impact

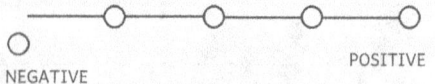

○——○——○——○
○
NEGATIVE   POSITIVE

Going Forward: CHANGE DOSAGE/ FREQUENCY ☐   TERMINATE USE ☐   CONTINUE USE ☐

MEDICAL ADVOCACY &
SELF-ADVOCACY GUIDE

*Asking the Right Questions
(And Knowing When to Get a Second Opinion)*

If Something Feels Off, Speak Up

If you feel your symptoms are being minimized or misunderstood, calmly redirect the conversation with evidence from your journal:

"I understand, but here are the patterns I've been tracking."

"This symptom has been consistent for weeks. What else can we explore?"

"What are the alternative explanations we haven't considered yet?"

Your documentation gives you strength and grounding.

Don't Be Afraid to Ask for a Second Opinion

Sometimes you need fresh eyes, a different perspective, or a doctor with specialized knowledge.

Needing a second opinion isn't rude. It isn't disrespectful. It isn't accusatory.

It is normal, appropriate, and often life-saving.

Say it clearly and confidently:

- "I'd like a second opinion to get more insight."
- "Can you refer me to a specialist who focuses on this type of symptom?"
- "I want to be as thorough as possible. A second opinion would help me feel more confident moving forward."

A good healthcare provider will support this—not shame it.

MEDICAL ADVOCACY &
SELF-ADVOCACY GUIDE

Asking the Right Questions
(And Knowing When to Get a Second Opinion)

Ask Questions That Get You Closer to Answers

"What are the possible causes of these symptoms?"

"What tests would help us narrow this down?"

"What do you think we should rule out first?"

"If these symptoms continue, what's the next step?"

"Could my medications be causing or worsening this?"

"Should I see a specialist about this?"

"What should I track more closely over the next few weeks?"

"What symptoms would require immediate care?"

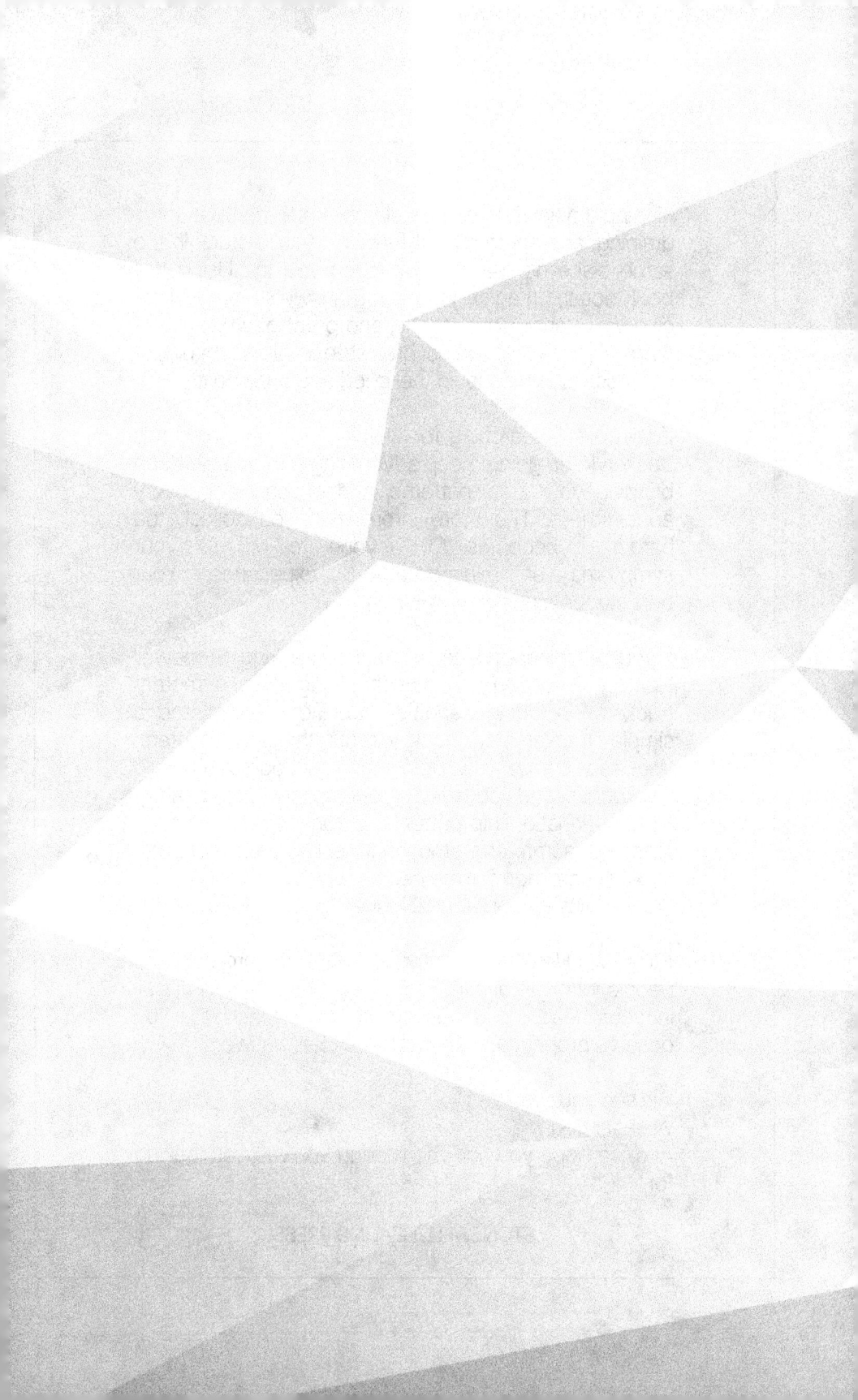

Finding a diagnosis is rarely simple. It can be frustrating, draining, and sometimes it feels like you're stuck in the same place no matter how much you try. Using this book doesn't magically give you answers—but it does give you clarity, consistency, and proof of what you've been living with. This is one step in a much bigger process, and you should feel good about taking it.

If you're still searching for answers after finishing this tracker, keep going. Keep advocating for yourself. Keep bringing your logs, patterns, and questions to every appointment. The more information you collect, the harder it becomes for anyone to dismiss your symptoms or minimize your experience. Your persistence matters.

If you need more space to continue tracking, Stonewell Healing Press offers additional diagnostic symptom trackers—including condition-specific versions and a simple "tracker-only" book without the extra content. We also create a wide range of trauma-informed workbooks and journals for people navigating family wounds, relationship patterns, chronic stress, burnout, medical trauma, and emotional healing. Everything we make is designed for the people who often go unheard in medical and mental-health spaces.

Stonewell Healing Press exists for the underdogs—the people who get overlooked, brushed off, or told "it's all in your head." You deserve to be listened to. You deserve proper care. You deserve clear answers.

We see you.
We hear you.
And we hope you find the healing you've been looking for.

STONEWELL HEALING PRESS

www.ingramcontent.com/pod-product-compliance
Lightning Source LLC
Chambersburg PA
CBHW062100270326
41931CB00013B/3155